Allied Health Professions

Patient Self Referral

A guide for therapists

Lesley Holdsworth

Clinical Effectiveness Co-ordinator
NHS Forth Valley
Stirling

and

Valerie Webster

Associate Dean (Quality)
School of Health and Social Care
Glasgow Caledonian University

Radcliffe Publishing
Oxford • Seattle

Radcliffe Publishing Ltd
18 Marcham Road
Abingdon
Oxon OX14 1AA
United Kingdom

www.radcliffe-oxford.com
Electronic catalogue and worldwide online ordering facility.

British Library Cataloguing in Publication Data

A catalogue record for this book is available from the British Library.

ISBN-10 1 84619 165 3
ISBN-13 978 1 84619 165 7

Typeset by Advance Typesetting Ltd, Oxford
Printed and bound by TJ International Ltd, Padstow, Cornwall

This book is dedicated to the very many physiotherapists throughout the UK and in particular the Scottish Physiotherapists Self Referral Study Group. On a personal level, we also dedicate these words to our 'Richards' and our girls, Claire, Rachel, Harriet, Kirsten and Nicole and thank them all for being so patient and understanding of us and forgiving our absences, we couldn't have done this without any of you!

Contents

About the authors

Lesley Holdsworth trained as a physiotherapist during the 1970s, working in a variety of settings throughout the UK. She has been working in Scotland since 1983 and developed an interest in service evaluation soon after arriving. National research fellowships and secondments during the late 1980s and early 1990s further developed this interest, particularly with regard to patient access and service provision. For the last 10 years she has been working with the full range of health professionals and is the lead for clinical effectiveness within NHS Forth Valley. Lesley was the co-founder and developer of the AHP National Clinical Effectiveness Networks that are now an integral part of NHS Quality Improvement Scotland. Most recently she has been a member of the Advisory Group of the National Framework for Service Change, a group charged by the Health Minister to put forward the vision for the NHS in Scotland and from which current policy is based. She also sits on a number of national and UK-wide policy and professional groups.

Despite having wide-ranging multiprofessional interests, Lesley has maintained strong professional links with physiotherapy, contributing to the work of the Chartered Society of Physiotherapy for which she was awarded a fellowship in 2005. This is also apparent in her major research interest, which, for the last 10 years, in conjunction with Valerie, has been in developing and evaluating the efficacy of patient self-referral systems in physiotherapy both nationally and internationally, about which she has widely published and presented. Lesley is currently working in collaboration with the CSP as an advisor to the Department of Health in England about patient self-referral services.

Valerie Webster also trained as a physiotherapist in the 1970s. Her interest in research related to practice and service evaluation developed whilst she was working within the NHS. It was during this time that she and Lesley first got together to work collaboratively comparing service provision in different health areas. Valerie moved into Higher Education in the early 1990s when she took up a post as a physiotherapy lecturer at Glasgow Caledonian University. Working in partnership she has lead the development of physiotherapy undergraduate and inter-professional postgraduate education programmes. She is currently Associate Dean (Quality) for the School of Health and Social Care and divides her time between this role and developing her research areas.

In conjunction with Lesley, her friend and colleague, a key area of research has for the past 10 years been developing and evaluating patient self-referral systems nationally and internationally. They have together presented and published widely on the subject. Currently she is working in collaboration with the Chartered Society of Physiotherapy as an advisor to the Department of Health in England about patient self-referral services.

Inter-professional learning and working forms the second strand of her practice and research interests. Her work in this area has led her, on behalf of two universities, to Chair a steering group developing inter-professional education and research involving nine different health and social care professions. She is a member of the Higher Education Academy and works closely with the professional body, NHS partners and the Quality Assurance Agency.

Introduction

Why write this guide?

We have been involved in introducing and evaluating patient self-referral physio-therapy services for over 10 years. What do we actually mean by patient self-referral? We have defined this as:

> ... a system of access which allows patients to refer themselves to a healthcare provider directly without having to see or be prompted by another healthcare practitioner. This relates to telephone, electronic technology or face-to-face services.

Over the last 10 years we have lost count of the enquiries we have fielded from all over the UK and from many other countries worldwide. We have been contacted by a wide range of healthcare providers: clinical staff from a variety of professions; therapists, nurses and doctors; service managers; professional bodies; and healthcare policy makers. They have raised all sorts of issues and, initially some-what surprising to us, has been the fact that regardless of profession, viewpoint, geographical setting and/or system of funding the questions have been the same.

The most frequently asked questions have been:

- 'Where do we start?'
- 'How do we go about it?'
- 'What do we need to do?'
- 'Are there any professional issues?'
- 'Are there specific training needs for staff?'
- 'How do we publicise it?'
- 'Will we able to cope with all the referrals?'
- 'What information should we collect?'
- 'How do we demonstrate impact?'

Purpose

We have tried to answer specific and general enquiries, but we always come back to the fact that the key determinant of success lies in how you prepare: doing your homework, really doing your homework and making 'critical friends'. This book is not intended to be an in-depth academic text about patient self-referral; rather, it is a practical guide that should help to take you 'relatively stress-free' through the very important key stages of preparation. We hope it will provide useful hints and tips to assist you in your decision-making and, if you decide to go ahead, will ensure you as successful and painless a transition as possible. The content is based on the knowledge we have gained through bitter (and sweet!) experience, and it is a representation of our personal views.

Who this book is for

This book is aimed at allied health professionals, but is also highly relevant to other healthcare practitioners.

It needs to be emphasised, however, that we are not aware of any professional body that does not support the concept of patient self-referral, but we need to point out that there are differences in what is acceptable in terms of individual professional scope of practice. For this reason, we advise readers who are seriously considering introducing patient self-referral *to establish as soon as possible what the key issues and boundaries are for their profession* to save any unnecessary effort. Once you have reviewed your Rules of Professional Conduct if you are still in any doubt your professional body will be able to provide advice.

Once the basis for patient self-referral has been established, however, irrespective of profession or service sector, the issues that need to be considered are just the same.

How to use this guide

The content of each part of the book is based on the questions that have been asked of us most frequently. We have tried to group them logically and in the order that you need to consider them in your preparation for introducing patient self-referral services. Each part aims to provide some of the answers but also poses for consideration other key issues that we have discovered through experience to be important. At the end of each part you will find a checklist of suggested actions to consider and a further reading list which relates to the topics covered. In addition to providing practical hints and top tips throughout the text, we also include suggested datasets and practical tools that we hope will aid you in being as fully prepared as possible.

Part I

Chapter 1

Background

Traditionally, within the UK and many other countries worldwide, patients gain access to therapy practitioners primarily through two channels:

- By referring themselves directly to private providers.
- By securing an onward referral from a doctor.

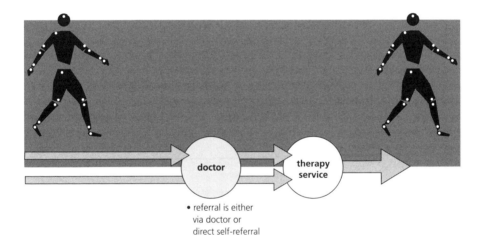

Before we start to consider the practicalities of introducing patient self-referral, it is useful to remember that private therapy practitioners all over the world have a long and successful track record of providing services to patients who refer themselves. They have developed approaches, processes and systems that ensure that patients referring themselves to their services are managed professionally, effectively and safely. Patient self-referral to the public funded system of healthcare provided within the UK is nowhere near as developed and we have much to learn from the experiences of our colleagues in the private sector.

Our work has been in developing physiotherapy patient self-referral services in the public funded sector and we draw from this experience throughout this text. It must be noted however that the issues, the healthcare policy context and structures in place are just as relevant to many other professions, irrespective of sector and location.

Tracing the progress of access to physiotherapy

Like many other therapy services, physiotherapy is a dynamic, developing profession. Since its inception over 100 years ago, it has evolved into a profession of autonomous highly skilled practitioners.

Introduction of open access

Many physiotherapists practising today will have no idea, let alone have experience, of a time in physiotherapy history when general practitioners (GPs) were not allowed to refer patients directly for outpatient physiotherapy. Before 1981, in all but a few locations, access to physiotherapy was only through hospital consultants, who, if they felt it appropriate, would refer the patient on. Restricted access like this also applied to many other allied health professions at the time – a practice that would be inconceivable today. The pressure to allow GPs access to physiotherapy, often referred to as 'open access', eventually resulted in a change in national UK policy in 1981, establishing open access as a universal right of GPs, as also happened at a similar time in a number of other countries globally.

Interestingly, a survey conducted by the Royal College of General Practitioners (RCGP) and the Chartered Society of Physiotherapy (CSP) 10 years later (in 1990) identified that there were areas of the UK where GPs still did not have open access. Despite this, during the 1980s and 1990s, referrals to physiotherapy across the UK increased significantly and by as much as fourfold in some locations.

Impact of introducing GP open access services

The increase in referrals over this time was attributed to successive government health policies that aimed to shift care away from hospital to primary care settings, to increase access to services and improve patients' experience of healthcare. These aims were primarily driven by a need to curb expenditure but were also a response to the rising consumerism in society. Patients became more knowledgeable and discerning about their healthcare options and more vocal at expressing their expectations.

Arguably, the government healthcare reform singularly most responsible for the increase in referrals to therapy services was the introduction of GP fund-holding in 1990. Fund-holding encouraged and allowed groups of GPs to use a devolved budget to purchase services on behalf of their patients. This had a dramatic effect on the number of referrals to therapy services. GPs recognised the value of these services for their patients and the value for money they represented.

Evaluations of open access services reported significant benefits for patients and services, identifying benefits such as improved patient outcomes and satisfaction, decreased service costs and decreased waiting times.

From open access to self-referral

The continued growth and perceived success of primary care-based services throughout the 1990s initiated the debate on locus of control and patient access. For the first time and from various sectors of healthcare, including patients, the wisdom of allowing doctors only to control access to healthcare provision was questioned.

This debate was also heavily influenced by the development of primary care teams: multi-professional teams composed of more than just doctors and nurses. Teams commonly consisted of other healthcare practitioners: pharmacists, podiatrists, physiotherapists and occupational therapists, for example. They worked more coherently with increased communication delivering more and more healthcare locally and away from hospital settings. The traditional hierarchy, which had been biased heavily towards medical leadership, was starting to erode (Figure 1.1). GPs working more closely with the wider team recognised their skills, expertise and ability to work autonomously. The debate about open access was frequently initiated by GPs who saw at first hand the benefits for patients in gaining speedy access to the most appropriate healthcare practitioner. From this developing confidence in the new world of primary care, the traditional 'gatekeeper' role of GPs began to be questioned.

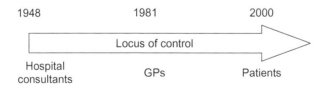

Figure 1.1 The change in locus of control.

The first reported examples of patient self-referral initiatives to emerge during the late 1990s were primarily nurse-led. They tended to consist of nurse-led clinics situated in both acute but mainly primary care settings where nurses worked autonomously providing services directly to patients with conditions such as diabetes, high blood pressure, asthma and so on. They were introduced to improve patient access to services and to provide continuity of care, but also as an answer to some of the workforce recruitment problems that GPs were facing at that time.

Reports of the evaluations of these services generated further interest and the potential relevance of patient self-referral to other therapy services, including physiotherapy, started to develop.

Chapter 2

Why consider patient self-referral?

As stated in Chapter 1, the evaluations of GP open access to therapy services identified significant benefits, which included:

- improved waiting times
- improved patient outcomes
- less treatment required
- greater patient satisfaction
- greater healthcare practitioner satisfaction
- increased cost-effectiveness.

With continued change in healthcare policy and an increasing emphasis on delivering high-quality services in the most appropriate location, services started to ask whether by introducing patient self-referral these benefits could be increased further.

As we moved into the new millennium an appetite to consider the real potential for patient self-referral to a number of therapy services began to emerge.

Current support for patient self-referral

What does the public think about self-referral?

The growth in societal consumerism since the 1980s has greatly influenced how healthcare is provided. Patients have become far more informed about healthcare options and have greater expectations, which they are more vocal at expressing. It appears that there is wide public support for easier access and in particular self-referral to a range of healthcare services.

Box 2.1 Recent examples of public support for patient self-referral to physiotherapy

---

Public polls undertaken in 2003 and 2004 by Mori and YouGov reported over 88% of respondents would prefer to refer themselves to physiotherapy than attend their GP first. (CSP, 2005)

What is the level of support from professional bodies?

Professional bodies representing professions such as dietetics, occupational therapy, optometry, physiotherapy, podiatry and nursing are supportive of the concept of patient self-referral. Patients' ability to self-refer is accepted practice in the private healthcare sector and the extension to include public-funded healthcare is seen as a change to NHS access arrangements rather than as a change in professional practice.

Cautionary point

Do ensure that your profession supports patient self-referral and that it is not considered an extension to scope of practice, as this has implications. Seek guidance from your professional body before progressing.

Is patient self-referral supported by healthcare policy?

We have already alluded to the fact that many of the changes in practice since 1990 have been driven by healthcare policy. The most recent government health policies from each of the UK member countries have continued to put primary care at the centre of the development of health services. Although tailored to the needs of each country, they consistently outline the intention to improve quality, achieve better, fairer access with increased flexibility, improve communication and reduce waiting times. They also emphasise that patient access and flexible delivery are important strands of the modern NHS.

Box 2.2 Recent example of healthcare policy support for patient self-referral to therapy services

In 2006, an English Department of Health policy document went so far as to identify the need for piloting and evaluation of self-referral services and particularly therapy services:

'self-referral to therapist services has the potential to increase patient satisfaction and save valuable GP time. In order to provide better access to a wider range of services, we will pilot and evaluate self-referral to physiotherapy ...' (DoH, 2006: 94)

The need to pilot and evaluate patient self-referral services was recognised because of the limited evidence on which to base service demand and the required resources. It was also an acknowledgement of a prevailing perception, voiced in some quarters, that removing medical control could result in increased referrals and demand for services that could not be met. It was not only an increase in referrals that was feared but also an increase in the overall costs to healthcare services as there was a train of thought that the relatively low cost of healthcare in the UK was because GPs acted as 'gate-keepers' to specialist services. More recently, the basis for this argument has been questioned.

It is true to say that successive government reforms, aimed to improve patient access and address workforce issues, have driven many of the developments in practice since 1990. The changes seen in the approach to healthcare delivery have also required individual healthcare practitioners to make changes in the way they have traditionally delivered care. Many of these changes have relied on autonomous ways of working, in a way and to an extent previously not experienced.

What is professional autonomy?

Professional autonomy can be summarised as the freedom to practise independently of external controls. Practising autonomously not only brings freedom of practice but also both professional and personal responsibility with increased accountability for the management of patients.

With regard to physiotherapy, the right to practise fully in this way was introduced in 1978. Physiotherapists were deemed capable of determining treatment, deciding when discharge was appropriate and accepting patients without a medical referral. This change had a considerable impact on private practitioners who, for the first time, were able to accept referrals from patients directly without a medical referral. Although some aspects of autonomous practice were introduced within the NHS, a medical referral continued to be required primarily because of fear that services would be overwhelmed if they opened their doors!

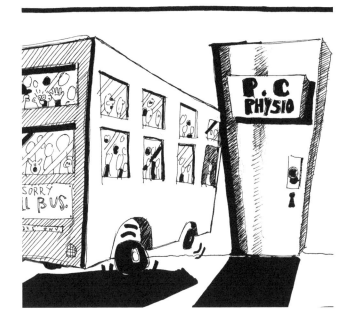

First point of contact practice – are we ready?

With responsibility comes accountability. If any profession wishes to assume the role of first point of contact practitioner it has to be prepared to assume the responsibilities which go with it. Traditionally, the first point of contact for patients seeking many services within the NHS has been the GP, who has for the most part controlled access by assuming the role of 'gatekeeper'. It is reasonable to assume that in a system where the doctor decides the most appropriate course of action, a proportion of staff may consciously or subconsciously abdicate some of their professional responsibility. This abdication is based on their belief that the GP will have screened the patient for potentially serious or complex problems and that the responsibility for doing this does not lie with them.

Managing all aspects of practice can be challenging and it has to be recognised that some healthcare practitioners may not be ready for this level of responsibility. Later on you will be asked to question if your staff have the skills and confidence to assume this role or, indeed, if they want to. It is crucial to the success of any patient self-referral service that staff members are willing and able to operate as first point of contact practitioners.

Chapter 3

Legal and professional considerations

> Q What are the legal issues, what do I need to know?

Legally, if you are working in the public sector, and patient self-referral is supported by your organisation, there are *no* additional legal considerations *provided* your scope of practice and level of autonomy permits patient self-referral.

In our experience, however, it is worth spending time discussing concerns with staff members as we have found that certain questions are raised consistently and they need to be clarified and assurance provided.

Other issues raised

A commonly raised concern relates to scope of practice and roles and responsibilities in systems of self-referral, a concern that is unfounded if your profession is permitted to accept patients without a medical referral. Some of the questions asked of us have included the following.

> Q Has my level of responsibility for the patient (known as 'duty of care') changed?

Practising in a service which permits patient self-referral should be no different professionally or legally to practising in a service where a doctor or other health professional referral is required. When a patient is received for assessment and/or treatment, a duty of care is established. This should be reflected in your Rules of Professional Conduct.

The relevant section for physiotherapy states:

> Physiotherapists have a responsibility to ensure that the therapeutic intervention is intended to be of benefit to the patient.
> (Rule 1.5)

A breach of duty of care or negligence occurs when there is failure to take reasonable care. This circumstance could occur in either referral system.

As we stressed before, it is essential that all staff involved are fully professionally developed and aware of their responsibilities in accepting this role. Systems of patient self-referral will require some therapy staff to think very differently.

Q What if someone with a serious problem or pathology is lying on the waiting list?

This concern has been voiced on a number of occasions over the years. This situation is possible so it is essential that whichever system is put in place you have a mechanism for reviewing referrals and that patients provide enough information for you to make an informed decision about their status.

Top tip

Having referral forms that patients complete, and a system for reviewing and triaging patients, can avoid this situation arising.

In our experience, how you receive your referrals and the information sought from patients during this process are crucial to reassuring staff. On many occasions, we have found that the quality and completeness of information provided by patients referring themselves is more enlightening than referrals from medical sources.

Examples of patient self-referral forms used in some physiotherapy services are included in the appendices. More can be found by visiting www.selfreferralphysioinfo.com.

Q Do I need to make any changes to the way I keep my patient records?

As in all areas of practice, it is both a professional and legal requirement to keep accurate patient records. In the case of self-referring patients, the therapy record may be the only record of the fact that the patient sought help for a problem. It goes without saying that *all* records should be accurate, detailed and up to date. In the rare case of a patient deciding to instigate proceedings against a healthcare practitioner, he or she has three years in which to do so, further highlighting the need for good-quality record-keeping.

Check that your current patient record-keeping guidance and standards include asking staff to provide written evidence of:

- assessment
- clinical reasoning and analysis of the patient's problem(s)
- clinical reasoning and evidence of rationale for treatment choice
- goals for treatment mutually agreed with patients
- discharge status and rationale
- additional issues of note and relevance
- key contact dates
- a legible signature.

See Part III of this book for further details.

Top tip

Courts tend to see a correlation between poor or inadequate record-keeping and poor quality standards of professionalism. This might lead them to question the credibility of the physiotherapist when considering a defendant's case. (CSP, 2005)

Q Will my professional liability insurance cover increase?
Q Does the department need enhanced insurance cover?

Professional bodies recommend that their members check the level and extent of vicarious responsibility at the start of their employment so they are fully aware of their cover.

Guidance provided by the Chartered Society of Physiotherapy (CSP), for example, states:

> It is important that members do not extend their scope of practice
> in such a way that is unknown or unacceptable to the employer.

Self-referral, although demanding certain professional attributes, is not (for physiotherapists at least) an extension of practice.

Top tip

As previously emphasised, you should ensure that self-referral is an accepted part of your profession's practice and that your organisation supports your plans for introducing patient self-referral services.

> **Q Do I need specific, informed consent from patients who self-refer?**

It could be argued that, as the patient has taken the initiative to refer him- or herself, consent is fully implied, possibly more so than when he or she is referred by a third party. This should not be taken for granted.

We identified in our work that a significant proportion of 'self-referring' patients were, in fact, referred at the suggestion of their GP and a truly autonomous decision was not taken by the patient. We have no reason to doubt that this practice will continue and you should be alerted to this.

It is expected that when obtaining consent from any patient sufficient information must be provided to allow informed consent to be provided. In addition, it should be made absolutely clear to patients who self-refer that they are being assessed and managed by a healthcare practitioner practising autonomously. In all other aspects of practice, obtaining and recording consent remains the same.

Some other questions

We have often been asked these questions and give the same answer each time.

> **Q Can children refer themselves to physiotherapy?**
> **Q What about patients who lack capacity to give their consent?**
> **Q What if a patient refuses treatment?**

The fact that these patients have self-referred makes them, or the way in which they are managed, no different than if they were referred from a medical source. The same rules apply.

What would be your response if these were medical referrals?

> **Top tips**
>
> • For many professions there are *no* additional legal or professional issues.
> • Make sure your organisation supports your service changes.
> • Ensure services are delivered in line with your professional body's 'Rules of Professional Conduct'.
> • Ensure that staff have the appropriate training, skills, expertise and are fully aware of their legal and professional standing.
> • Apply the same professional standards regardless of how patients are referred.

Practising as a 'first point of contact practitioner' may be a new concept for some of your staff so it is well worth taking the time to highlight to them the following points.

Confidence

Some therapists may feel wary of assuming a role when the perceived 'safety net' of screening traditionally undertaken by the referring doctor has been removed. With no 'gate keeper' there is always the chance that potentially very complex and inappropriate cases may refer themselves.

It is essential that staff involved are experienced enough to recognise the breadth and depth of their practice and have the confidence to deal with all aspects of patient management, including knowing when their professional expertise is not the most appropriate course of action.

Confidence is also required when interacting with the other members of the healthcare team whether promoting the benefits of self-referral or discussing aspects of patient management.

Top tips

- Clarify professional and legal issues with your staff at the outset.
- Assess if your staff are experienced enough to recognise the breadth and depth of practice needed.
- Do they have the confidence to deal with all aspects of patient management?
- Do they have the confidence to interact with other members of the healthcare team.
- Ensure that your staff members feel supported through this period of transition.

Scope of practice

Staff members need to be fully aware of their scope of practice and that the potential exists for this to be challenged when patients self-refer. Discuss with GPs and other potential referrers the scope and operation of your service.

Top tip

Ensure that clinical staff and potential referrers to your service are fully informed and aware of your professional scope of practice.

Communication

As in most aspects of healthcare delivery, effective communication is funda-
mental to optimum care. Being able to communicate with patients and
other healthcare practitioners is crucial. Strong formal links will be needed.

We need to recognise that, in some instances, self-referring patients may
be more demanding or indeed more anxious, which could be a challenge for
some staff. Ensure that staff members are adequately developed professionally to manage diverse, 'unscreened' caseloads effectively.

Top tips

- Ensure that staff members have had adequate professional development and are encouraged to develop their communication skills.
- Listen carefully to patients.
- Establish effective communication links between your staff and
  other healthcare practitioners.
- Use feedback from service users and other healthcare practitioners
  to inform staff development and identify needs.

Critical thinking

It seems too obvious to include critical thinking as essential to the success of
self-referral, but it is. Practising autonomously requires highly developed
critical thinking skills. Although the majority of clinical staff members are
now trained in approaching issues in this way, not all staff may be so
confident and competent.

Patient self-referral requires therapists to reflect on and evaluate their
practice critically to be able to define their own scope of practice and identify
their learning needs at any stage in their development.

Top tip

Ensure that staff members are aware of the professional requirements
associated with self-referral and that they have the capacity to:

- practise autonomously
- self-regulate
- demonstrate openness, honesty and transparency in practice
- take responsibility and be accountable for all aspects of practice.

The two most frequently asked questions about grades of staff

Q What about juniors?
Q What about students?

Guidelines for supporting and supervising newly qualified staff remain unchanged. The points noted previously regarding scope of practice, communication and confidence apply to all grades of staff. To ensure success, however, newly qualified staff should clearly understand the role of their mentor and the limits of their own competence and capability. Although newly qualified members of many professions are autonomous on qualification, it is accepted that competence and capability develop with time. The point when a member of staff is fully ready to assume the role of first point of contact without direct support will vary from individual to individual.

As far as students are concerned, again, nothing changes. In the traditional referral system student caseloads and activity are monitored and directed by more senior staff who are ultimately responsible for the patient. With self-referring patients this remains unchanged. In our experience information provided by self-referral patients has, in many instances, been more detailed and relevant to their condition than some of the information provided via third-party referrals.

By engaging students in this developing area of practice we are preparing them more fully for practice on qualification. In addition, engaging students allows them to see how professional, responsible and accountable they will need to be if they are to practise successfully in a modern health service.

Top tip

Successfully engaging staff is assisted by:

- all staff feeling supported
- newly qualified or inexperienced staff being provided with additional guidance and support
- providing clear guidance as to when assistance should be sought
- clarifying scope of practice
- embedding ongoing review and evaluation
- providing guidance and support to develop communication and confidence
- developing a culture of openness and honesty.

Do your staff members want to do this? Are you sure?

There is no point in introducing services that are not supported by the staff members who are expected to deliver them. In our experience, enlisting staff who feel ready and able to act as first point of contact practitioners is the only way forwards. As with all major changes to practice, having local champions will pay dividends and facilitate the whole process.

Cautionary point

Staff members who lack confidence or have misgivings about this development not only undermine their own practice but may inadvertently convey these feelings to patients – with negative consequences.

Top tips

- Support and encourage your staff.
- Take time to prepare them fully.
- Do not assume that all staff will happily take on this role.
- Address issues of accountability, responsibility, confidence and/or communication head on.
- Identify and court your champions.

By now you should have an idea of why patient self-referral has developed. You should also be quite clear of your own profession's legal and professional stance in relation to a range of service provision options, including patient self-referral.

There are many examples of service developments, all with the similar aim of improving patient access to healthcare, but when they are examined more closely, are actually very different.

It is often assumed when we use certain labels to describe our services that their meaning will be understood by all. In our experience this is not always the case. In this book we have referred to 'patient self-referral' consistently, but what exactly do we mean and why did we choose to use this phrase to describe the service offered?

Chapter 4

What do we mean by patient self-referral?

At the start of this book, we provided the definition of patient self-referral we use:

> Patient self-referral is a system of access that allows patients to refer themselves to a healthcare service provider directly, without having to see or be prompted by another healthcare practitioner. This relates to telephone, electronic technology or face-to-face services.

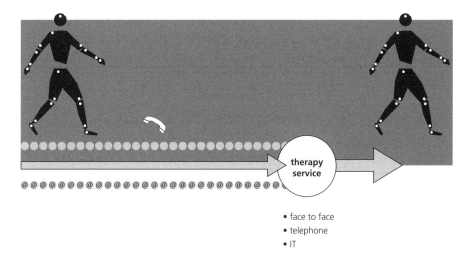

- face to face
- telephone
- IT

So what's in a name?

Well, actually quite a lot. When we first started introducing patient self-referral physiotherapy services in the mid-1990s, we initially called these services 'direct access services' or 'Physiotherapy Direct'. A logical choice of name that quite transparently described what was being offered: patients had direct access themselves, or did it? We continued to refer to these services in this way for the next five years or so, but, in 2003, we made the deliberate decision to stop using these terms for a number of reasons.

Why consider changing?

As interest grew in the concept of physiotherapy self-referral schemes, other physiotherapy services started to emerge throughout the UK. Many called themselves 'direct access' services, but, on closer examination, these proved to be very different indeed in terms of how patients actually accessed them. We have always been zealously committed to rigorously evaluating the impact of patient self-referral to provide a credible view of its overall efficacy. The subsequent emergence of services that were fundamentally very different but which referred to themselves in the same way, we felt, was not only confusing to patients, the wider public and clinical staff but would 'muddy' any attempt to compare between sites into the future.

How were the services different?

We found examples of direct access services which had introduced a system that allowed patients to refer themselves, but only after being suggested they do so by another healthcare practitioner.

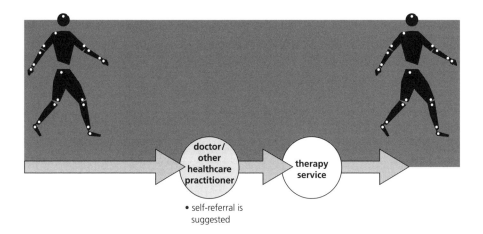

In these cases, the onus is placed on patients to make the effort to arrange appointments themselves. This has two main benefits. First, it removes the paperwork associated with referral from the system, very popular with GPs especially, and, second, it ensures that only those who are motivated refer themselves. What is not known, however, is whether these patients would have instigated this course of action if left to their own devices.

Although offering advantages for both patients and referrers, these services are not examples of 'true' self-referral. They are efforts, undoubtedly positive efforts, to widen access and streamline the referral process.

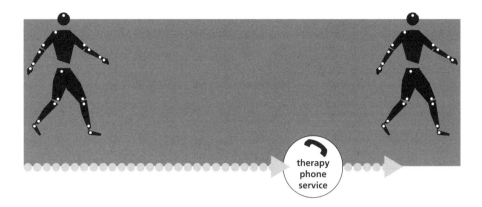

Other services operated telephone access, having first publicised themselves to patients in different ways. Quite often, such services offered front-line advice and then onwards referral if indicated.

We also came across examples of services describing themselves as 'direct access' services which turned out to be different again. These are services that allow patients, after being discharged, to re-refer themselves directly at any time in the future if they feel this is required. Many podiatry and speech and language services, for example, provide their services in this way. What differentiates these types of services from others is the fact that patients need a formal referral to gain access to the service in the first place before they can exercise any right to refer themselves further.

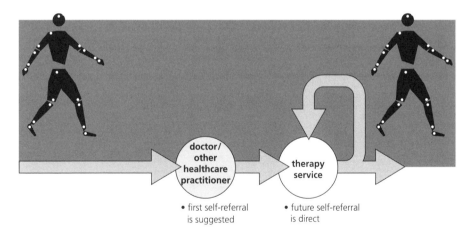

Our view is that these types of services, although highly appropriate, should not be confused with those which offer access to patients who have made the decision to refer themselves without being prompted by other health-care practitioners: thus acting in a truly autonomous manner.

Direct access: from whose perspective?

Our concerns grew over time. When discussing the issue with GPs, for example, the doctors would often retort that they already had direct access to physiotherapy, and, from their perspective, they did. This lack of clarity also extended to the policy makers, who were unclear as to exactly what constituted a 'direct access' service. We were party to discussions on a number of occasions between physiotherapists who thought they were offering similar services just because they had the same title when, in fact, they were very different. These are good examples of the confused use of terms commonly found in all aspects of healthcare.

Our solution

We were becoming more and more concerned about the lack of clarity and perspective. What must it be like as a potential user of services? We took the decision to use a different name, to make patients and their decision-making clearly as the focus and from that time we have referred to these services simply as 'patient self-referral services'. We found using this title removed ambiguity and distinguishes these services from the variety of other options available.

So that is our story, but we urge others to think seriously about this. Ensure that whatever you decide to call your service, its title is a true reflection of what is being provided, and consider the issue from a number of perspectives, and particularly from that of the wider public. There is nothing wrong and, indeed, it could even be said to be professionally responsible to look at a variety of ways to widen access to services for the benefit of users and providers. We have come to realise, however, how very important it is to apply consistent terminology to avoid confusion for patients and ensure that we are not talking about apples when we really mean pears or even bananas!

Top tips

- Check out what others are calling their services and what they actually provide or deliver.
- Ensure that the title of your service truly reflects what it is providing.
- Make clear to patients, staff and other stakeholders exactly what your service provides.
- Test out your ideas with a variety of audiences, including potential service users, before making a definitive decision.
- Keep key messages simple and clear.

Chapter 5

Checklist

You should now complete this checklist before you move on to Part II. Missing out key aspects of preparation at this stage may severely hamper your ability to progress.

Checklist I

- I have reviewed and now understand the guidance provided by my professional body in relation to patient self-referral. ☐
- My organisation supports the concept of my service introducing patient self-referral. ☐
- I have reviewed and now understand relevant policy documents that may have implications for my service. ☐
- I have reviewed and am now aware of the key evidence sources regarding patient self-referral. ☐
- I understand the legal and professional aspects as they apply to patient self-referral and my service. ☐
- I have developed a specific communications strategy that ensures formal links are made within and between my service and other stakeholders, including key referral sources. ☐
- My staff understands the legal and professional aspects as they apply to patient self-referral and the service. ☐
- I have sought out services users and patient advocacy groups to seek involvement in any developments. ☐
- I have made the effort to find out what other kinds of patient self-referral services are being delivered locally and wider. ☐
- I understand the importance of calling the patient self-referral service by a clear and unambiguous title. ☐

Chapter 6

Useful websites

Allied health professions: professional body websites:

- Association of Professional Music Therapists (www.apmt.org)
- British Association of Art Therapists (www.baat.org)
- British Association of Drama Therapists (www.badth.org.uk)
- British and Irish Orthoptic Society (www.orthoptics.org.uk)
- British Association of Prosthetics and Orthotists (www.bapo.org)
- British Dietetic Association (www.bda.uk.com)
- Chartered Society of Physiotherapy (www.csp.org)
- College of Occupational Therapists (www.cot.org)
- Royal College of Speech and Language Therapists (www.rcslt.org)
- Society and College of Radiographers (www.sor.org)
- Society of Chiropodists and Podiatrists (www.feetforlife.org)

Resource or information packs produced by each of the professional bodies are a great source for clarifying issues such as scope of practice, legal issues and so forth. Most are available via their members' website.

Other useful websites include the following:

- www.dh.gov.uk
- www.scotland.gov.uk
- www.wales.gov.uk
- www.dhsspsni.gov.uk
- www.scotland.gov.uk/health/cmo/incapacity.acltoc.asp
- www.opsi.gov.uk/ACTS
- www.statistics.gov.uk
- www.wales.gov.uk/keypubstatisticsforwales/content/publication/
- www.nisra.gov.uk

Chapter 7

Further reading

Akpala CO, Curran AP and Simpson J (1988) Physiotherapy in general practice: patterns of utilisation. *Public Health*. **102**: 263–8.

Coulter A (1998) Managing demand: managing demand at the interface between primary care and secondary care. *BMJ*. **316**: 1974–6.

Department of Health (1990) National Health Service and Community Care Act. HMSO, London.

Department of Health (2000) *The NHS Plan: a plan for investment, a plan for reform*. DoH, London.

Department of Health (2002) *Delivering the NHS Plan*. DoH, London.

Department of Health (2006) *Our Health, Our Care, Our Say, A New Direction for Community Services*. DoH, London.

Department of Health and Social Security (1972) Statement by the committee on the Standing Medical Advisory Committee (Turnbridge Report). HMSO, London.

Department of Health and Social Security (1977) Health service development: relationship between the medical and remedial professions. *Health Circular* HC[0](77):33.

Department of Health and Social Security (1981) *Orthopaedic Services: waiting time for outpatient appointments and inpatient treatment* (Duthie Report). HMSO, London.

Dowling S (1996) Nurses taking on junior doctors' work: a confusion of accountability. *BMJ*. **312**: 1211–14.

England T (1997) Personal paper: medicine in the 1990s needs a team approach. *BMJ*. **314**: 661–3.

Eve R, Gerrish K, Mares P, Metcalf H and Munro J (2001) *More than One Way to Skin a Cat. Building Capacity in Primary Care to Reduce Pressure on Hospitals*. Centre for Innovation in Primary Care (www.innovate.org.uk/frameset.asp?Link=DM).

Fordham R and Hodkinson C (1998) *A Cost Benefit Analysis of Open Access to Physiotherapy for GPs*. Discussion Paper 29. Centre for Health Economics, Health Economics Consortium, University of York.

Forrest C (2003) Primary care gatekeeping and referrals: effective filter or failed experiment? *BMJ*. **326**: 692–5.

Galley P (1977) Physiotherapists as first contact practitioners. *Physiotherapy*. **63**: 246–8.

Groves T (1999) Reforming British primary care (again). *BMJ*. **318**: 747–8.

Holdsworth L, Webster V and McFadyen A (2004) Direct access to physiotherapy in primary care: now – and into the future? *Physiotherapy*. **90**: 64–72.

Kinnersley P, Anderson E, Part K *et al.* (2000) Randomised controlled trial of nurse practitioner versus general practitioner care for patients requesting 'same day' consultations in primary care. *BMJ*. **320**: 1043–8.

Minns C and Bithell C (1998) Musculoskeletal physiotherapy in general practice fundholding practices. *Physiotherapy*. **84**: 84–92.

Munro J, Nicholl J, O'Cathain A *et al.* (2000) Impact of NHS Direct on demand for immediate care: observational study. *BMJ*. **321**: 150–3.

McKinnon M, Townsend J and Walker Z (1999) Primary care: past and future. *Health Services Management Research*. **12**: 143–8.

O'Cathain A, Munro J, Nicholl J *et al.* (2000) How helpful is NHS Direct? Postal survey of callers. *BMJ*. **320**: 1035.

O'Cathain A, Froggett M and Taylor MP (1995) General practice based physiotherapy: its use and effect on referrals to hospital orthopaedics and rheumatology outpatient departments. *Br J Gen Pract*. **45**: 352–4.

Rayner C (1999) Stuff and nonsense. *Nursing Standard*. **13**: 22–3.

Robert G and Stevens A (1997) Should general practitioners refer patients directly to physical therapists? *Br J Gen Pract*. **47**: 314–18.

Scottish Executive (2000) *Partnership for Care*. Scotland's Health White Paper. HMSO, Edinburgh (www.scotland.gov.uk/library3/health/ronh.pdf).

Scottish Executive (2002) *Building on Success – Future Directions for the Allied Health Professions in Scotland* (www.scotland.gov.uk/Publications/2002/06/14963/7835).

Scottish Executive (2003) *Rebuilding our National Health Service. A Plan for Action. A Plan for Change* (www.scotland.gov.uk/library5/health/pfcs.pdf).

Scottish Executive (2004) *Fair to All, Personal to Each, the Next Steps for NHS Scotland* (www.scotland.gov.uk/Publications/2004/12/20400/48699).

Scottish Executive (2005) *Delivering for Health Scotland* (www.scotland.gov.uk/Publications/2005/11/02102635/26356).

Scottish Office (1997) *Designed to Care: renewing the National Health Service in Scotland* (www.scotland.gov.uk).

Venning P, Durie A, Roland, M *et al.* (2000) Randomised controlled trial comparing cost effectiveness of general practitioners and nurse practitioners in primary care. *BMJ*. **320**: 1048–53.

Welsh Assembly (2001) *Improving Health in Wales: a plan for the NHS and its partners*. DoH, Cardiff.

Welsh Assembly (2002) *Improving Health in Wales: from plan to action*. DoH, Cardiff.

Welsh Assembly (2005) *Designed for Life: creating a world class health and social care for Wales in the 21st century*. DoH, Cardiff.

Wilkinson J (1997) Developing a concept analysis of autonomy in nursing practice. *Br J Nurse*. **6**: 703–807.

Part II

Chapter 8

Before you start

The most important tip we can give anyone who asks about how to introduce patient self-referral services is that, in our experience, preparation is the key to success, and this means doing your homework. A question often asked is this.

Q Where do I start?

Before you even think of getting started, or deciding which kind of patient self-referral system is right for you, there are some basic pieces of homework you need to do. These involve gathering key information about your population, your service and your critical friends.

Chapter 9

Know your population

How much do you really know about the population your service covers? We have found that the level of awareness varies enormously from site to site. Can you reply to the following statements?

- I know the size of the population my service covers.
- I know what proportion of the population live in urban, semi-rural or rural areas.
- I know exactly the deprivation indices of each area.
- I know the gender, age and ethnic breakdown of the population and if this differs throughout the area.
- I know if the profile and size of the population has changed over the last three years.

Why is it important to know this?

It is known that the demand for healthcare provision differs throughout the country and also within individual regions. The available evidence, however, relates mainly to medical services and although we have no cause to believe that this should be any different for therapy services, the information about these services is not so robust.

With regard to physiotherapy, the recently reported national trial of patient self-referral identified that there are differences in the average number of referrals to be expected in locations which differ in terms of their geography and, to some extent, their level of deprivation. Other work we have undertaken has also identified that, in some settings, the demand for physiotherapy was directly linked to an increased older population, an issue that will be just as appropriate to other healthcare service providers.

Top tip

A good starting point is to track down and collate this information. It should be relatively easy to do but if you are experiencing difficulties, strategic health boards or regions can often provide you with this information. Public health departments are also a very good source of information.

Although the rate of patient self-referral into the future is impossible to predict, having up-to-date information about your population will make any predictions much more accurate.

Chapter 10

Know your service

For the same reasons that it is important to know your population, you also have to have an intimate knowledge of your service. How much do you really know? Can you provide yearly statistics in answer to the following questions?

- What is the referral rate to your service, i.e. do you know how many new patients you see?
- Can you express this as a proportion per 1000 of the population? (We explain this later in this section.)
- Can you provide a breakdown of referral rates per individual site?
- Can you provide a breakdown of exactly where all these new patients came from, i.e. do you know the exact sources: GPs, consultants, other sources, etc.?
- Do you know what investigations or drugs these new patients had or were prescribed?
- Do you know what proportion is classed as appropriate?
- Do you have a waiting list? If so, how long is it? Does it vary and, if so, to what extent?
- Can you provide a breakdown of the profile of your patients? (By age, gender, condition, contacts, outcomes?)
- Do you have patient employment or work absence statistics?
- Do you know how many patients fail to attend for their first appointment or do not fully complete their course of treatment?
- Do you know what happens to patients after they are discharged?
- Do you know how many patients proceed for secondary referral, surgery or other management options?
- Do you know exactly where your service is, provided in terms of whole-time equivalents and sessions?
- Do you know exactly what your staffing complement is, expressed as whole-time equivalents per grade?
- Do you know how many students your service accommodates?
- Do you know what patients think about your service?

As before, we cannot emphasise strongly enough how important this information is to you. It will form the backbone of your baseline data, which is vital to make any credible judgement of impact into the future.

Getting hold of this information should not pose too much difficulty, but, if historically you have not been used to collecting certain types of information or data (patient employment information, for example), it may prove impossible to do retrospectively.

Having some information, however, is better than having no information. There is nothing to stop you collecting this information prospectively. This could be done in parallel with making your general preparations for introducing patient self-referral over a short period of time – three months, for example.

Top tips

- Get hold of as much information as you can.
- Having some information is better than having no information.
- Consider a short prospective data collection project to assist with accurate baseline data.
- Seek out the information analyst in your organisation for some help or reassurance with verifying your data.
- You need baseline data from which to make a credible judgement of the impact introducing patient self-referral has had.

Chapter 11

What kind of patient self-referral service is right for you?

You now should have gathered information about the population you serve and the service that is currently delivered. It is now time to consider exactly which kind of patient self-referral service is right for your overall needs.

Not only are there different ways in which patients can access your service, either directly or indirectly themselves or by being referred by another healthcare practitioner, there are also different ways of providing patient self-referral services. We described some of these in Part I. Your next step is to work out which one is for you. Before you do that, however:

- Have you gathered enough information about the options available to you?
- Have you contacted or visited other self-referral sites to hear or see at first hand what their experience has been?

By their nature, services vary depending on location, staffing, ethnicity, socio-economic factors as well as other locally determined factors. Not all patients wish or indeed have the confidence to refer themselves. What is very clear, however, is that whatever kind of patient self-referral service you decide on you will have to ensure that it is offered as an *additional* way of gaining access to your service not as the *only* one.

Top tips

- Take the time and effort to find out how others have introduced self-referral: ask them for their top tips! Don't re-invent the wheel; be prepared to learn from the mistakes of others! Not sure how to find 'others'? Try contacting your professional body; put a call out in your professional journal for information. Actively elicit information.
- You need an approach that suits your healthcare situation, not forgetting the resources to implement and sustain it.

What are the options available?

Here, we have tried to provide a description of a range of options that are potentially available to you. They represent a summary of the some of the examples we have come across in our travels around the UK and internationally. This is not an exhaustive list and there may be other approaches not included. For example, we are aware of a system under development that uses the internet to take referrals and provide first-line advice to patients. This is still under development but you should keep an open mind to options that are emerging all the time.

We have classified the systems under the following headings.

- Telephone systems, for:
  - advice
  - assessment and management decisions (triage)
  - call back
  - self-referral
  - appointment allocation.
- Face-to-face services, for:
  - drop-in clinics
  - managed waiting list approach.

Before implementing any service you must identify which system or blend of systems you intend to develop. The resources you require will depend on the system(s) you choose. This might seem very obvious but unless you have established that you have all the elements in place, you are heading for disaster.

Telephone systems

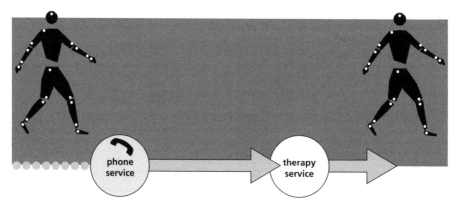

- screening or advice

Q **What type of service can be delivered over the telephone?**

Telephones are being used more and more to offer patients easy access to a range of services. Whether you intend to use a telephone system that allows patients to contact you directly for advice, assessment, management decision and prioritisation (triage), treatment options or to allocate appointments, consider the following points before proceeding.

Is a telephone option realistic bearing in mind your population?

Do you have a high ethnically diverse population, some of whom may be disadvantaged by such a system? This does not preclude you from introducing a telephone system but you also need to provide alternatives for this sector of your population.

The purpose of your service

Is it just for issuing appointments or for providing triage or advice? This will give an indication of how many lines you will need and who is needed to run the service. The greater level of service you offer, the more sophisticated a set up you will need.

Are there dedicated telephone lines available?

One telephone line is not likely to provide the required level of access for patients, and particularly so for larger populations. If you have an answering machine for times when the system isn't manned, how are you going to deal with messages? Have you the space for a call centre and work stations? For how long each day will telephones be manned? In reality, it is not worth introducing such a system if you cannot operate it at the times when patients will want to access it. Consider the impact of holidays and sickness. What is your back up plan? Consider whether evenings and or weekends are to be included in your plans.

Will all staff be involved?

If not which staff members will operate the telephones; develop firm and transparent criteria for selection. For how long are staff members expected to operate the telephones as a proportion of their working week? What arrangements have you made to provide staff with access to assistance with problematic calls? Even experienced staff may need to discuss complex cases. What training will be provided to staff? Are they provided with condition-specific algorithms or protocols to aid consistency in decision-making and service audit?

Do you need to be able to send out supporting information or advice to patients?

If so, do you have the appropriate high-quality evidence-based advice sheets or other health promotion material? How will you maintain your stock and ensure its ongoing quality?

Telephone systems and computers

If you intend to use a telephone system in conjunction with a computerised system to aid decision-making or patient administration, you will also have to consider the following.

- Is there currently a reliable server or information technology system?
- Before developing your own computer triage system look at the available validated options. There are an increasing number coming on the market, based on tried and tested algorithms, which should meet your needs and save you a lot of time and effort. They may require some local adaptation
- Do you have patient advice and health promotion material in an electronic format accessible on the system you are working?

An experience to learn from

A service in England introduced a telephone triage system serving a population of 50 000 people. It experienced significant problems due to its limited opening hours and the fact that it was manned by only one healthcare practitioner each morning between 9.30 am and 12 noon. Patients became very frustrated with not being able to get through and the service had to be abandoned causing loss of public confidence in their service.

Top tips

Consider your population.

- Certain sectors may have a difficulty in communicating adequately over the telephone?
- If there are specific language barriers, identify who will translate patient information into the key languages and formats required, and how this is to be resourced.
- Ensure that patients have ways of accessing your service other than by telephone.

Face-to-face services

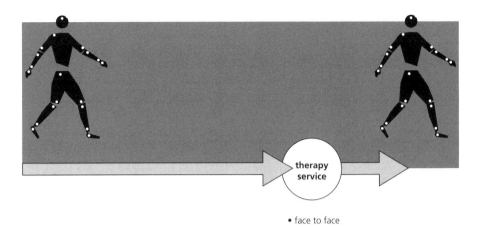

• face to face

The majority of therapy-led patient self-referral services currently operating in the UK NHS still involve a high level of face-to-face contact.

Patient self-referral should not provide preferential access for some patients. Irrespective of whether patients are referred by their GP or healthcare practitioner or refer themselves they should be treated equally at all stages in their management, including how long they wait to be seen and the treatment they receive. As said previously, patients (and other healthcare practitioners) may assume that patient self-referral means immediate access or a fast-track route to services. The principles on which you triage your waiting list should be applied consistently, regardless of mode of access. It is essential that the basis on which you manage your patient list is clearly understood by all clinical staff, patients and referring sources.

Providing face-to-face self-referral services should be developed with these principles in mind; remember, all you are doing is widening access to your services.

Some services have introduced 'drop-in clinics', which permit patients to turn up at an allotted time and be seen by a healthcare practitioner. Others have adopted a managed waiting list approach, where patients are allocated appointments in strict succession or based on how urgent their problem is perceived to be, usually judged from the referral information.

When considering what kind of approach to adopt, you might want to think about the following issues.

Drop-in clinics: key questions
What is the purpose of the clinic?

Do you plan to assess patients, offer advice, treat, arrange future physiotherapy or any combination of these approaches? Be clear about its purpose.

Do you have any idea of the potential demand?

This could influence:

- Where the clinic will be held – remember accessibility.
- Whether the clinic will be open to GP referrals as well as self-referrals – it is difficult to restrict access to just one sector.
- Waiting room accommodation.
- How often the clinic will be run.
- What times it will operate.
- How it will be staffed – skill mix, administrative support?
- What you will do with patients who need to be referred to their GP or other healthcare practitioner either routinely or on an urgent basis?
- How you will deal with patients who are turned away if the clinic is full?

Top tips

- It is possibly advisable to put your 'toe in the water' in the first instance and pilot your drop-in clinic to establish demand and working arrangements.
- Be clear about the purpose of the clinic and the basis on which it operates: clarify with staff, service users and potential referrers.

The managed waiting list approach

This is usually the much more controllable option, particularly in the early stages when you may be unsure of the immediate impact of offering patients the ability to self-refer to your service. The key considerations for this option include the following.

- Ensure that patients, irrespective of source of referral, are placed on the waiting list in the same way.
- Have criteria for managing your waiting list, which may or may not offer preferential access to prioritised categories of patients: more urgent conditions or the working population, for example.
- Set explicit definitions for your criteria and their level of priority, i.e. what does *urgent* actually mean? Are these patients to be offered the first available appointment? Make sure your categories are based on sound criteria and are communicated to, and understood by, all staff, patients and referrers.

Top tips

- Find out from other services their top tips and things to avoid!
- Marry your choice of approach to your population and service.
- More than one system can be introduced.
- Telephones are versatile and can be used in a number of ways.
- Self-referral does not mean the same as immediate or preferential access.

Chapter 12

The most frequently asked questions

Referral numbers

Without a doubt, the most frequently asked question of all relates to referrals, or rather the impact that introducing patient self-referral will have on the viability of a service.

It stems from a fear that we have been 'protected' in the past by GPs acting as gatekeepers to our services. The perception has been that GPs have prevented services from being overwhelmed by thousands of patients who, given half a chance, would beat their way to our door and not all of them appropriately!

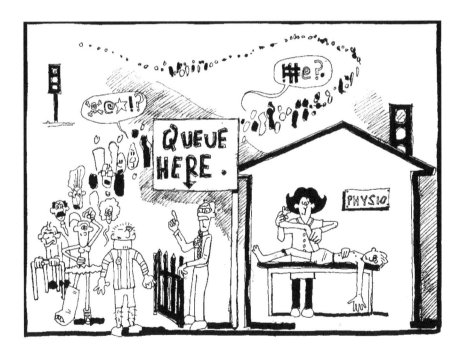

The fear of being overwhelmed has been prominent in hindering the development of patient self-referral services: a fear largely based on supposition but fuelled by the increasing rate of referral to a range of healthcare services over the last decade or so. More recent government health policies in the UK and globally have started to challenge this concept, promoting greater patient choice and widening access in the spirit of efficiency.

But longstanding traditions and a level of comfort are not so easy to dispel. In acknowledging this fear, people have been asking questions.

Q Will my service be able to cope?

In our experience, most services have coped extremely well.

In the recently reported national trial of patient self-referral to physiotherapy, less than 20% of sites experienced any increase in the overall number of referrals to their service above that found nationally. Those that did had one thing in common, a history of under-provision, that is, they had not previously been providing a level of service which was in line with the national averages identified for their location and level of deprivation.

An experience to learn from

While preparing to introduce patient self-referral, a service realised that one of its referral sources, a general practice, had been historically under-referring patients compared to other sources for many years. Staff were concerned about the possible effect on their service. Their concerns were well-founded and they experienced a significant increase in the number of overall referrals once patients became aware that they could refer themselves. You need to be prepared to review the resources available to meet potential demand.

Within the UK, it is fair to say that identifying and reporting referral trends accurately has not been a feature of healthcare services. Historically, services have tended to base their reporting on the number of new patients over a given time period alone without reference to other issues, and possibly for good reason as the debate has always centred on current service provision and not actual need.

For example, would it be really surprising if there had been a 10% increase in the number of annual referrals to a service if the community it served had increased its overall population during that time? Or, in a community which had built three new elderly care homes attracting in excess of 1000 older people to the area? How many services would know or report their activity in such a way?

> Q Is there any way I can anticipate the impact of introducing patient self-referral on the number of referrals to my service?

A much more accurate way of monitoring the referral rate is to express the number of referrals a service receives annually as a proportion of the population it serves. The most common currency used within healthcare throughout the UK for any type of referral is the proportion per 1000 of the overall population.

> Q How do I calculate my referral rate as a proportion per thousand?

In response, we have developed a 'tool' which will take the reader through this calculation. It can be found in Appendix V. We recommend that for accuracy, you carry out this calculation using the last three years of service data and find your average. This will then ensure that any annual discrepancies occurring due to extenuating circumstances are evened out: changes in referral sources, service delivery, staffing ratios and so on.

> **Top tip**
>
> Although originally developed for physiotherapy use, the referral calculator tool can be used by any service. It will still allow you to calculate your referral rate per 1000 and apply that to your geographical setting. In the absence of nationally available referral rates to your profession, we recommend that you ask your colleagues in differing regions to also undertake this calculation and then you could share your findings.

In parallel, we also advise that you check on the overall population of your catchment area for the same time period.

> Q What is a catchment area?

Services are generally provided to a population who live within a specified geographical area commonly referred to as a 'catchment area'. The dynamics of catchment areas and therefore the implications for healthcare service delivery can change with time. It is important that you keep abreast of changes on an ongoing basis.

You might want to keep on top of changes, such as the following.

- Have there been any major housing developments?
- Has the overall population increased or declined?
- Have the demographics changed?

Any of these changes will have potential implications for your service.

Q What about overlapping catchment areas?

It is essential that you are aware of where there are overlaps in your catchment area. Why? If you introduce a change that is perceived to improve access, then patients traditionally referred to other services may choose to refer themselves to your service, increasing demand on your resources. This is more likely to happen in urban rather than rural areas but not always!

You will need to consider how you will manage this. For example, what about the potential demand from patients who live outside your area but work locally?

National referral rates to therapy services

There is a distinct lack of reliable information about national referral rates to individual therapy services or even by region. In Scotland, there have been two significant pieces of recent work that have provided, for the first time, a national perspective. This information may be of use to you in your considerations. The key sources of this information are:

- National Multicentred Trial of Patient Self-referral to Physiotherapy (2003–05).
- National Allied Health Professions (AHP) Census results (2005).

As part of the national trial of self-referral to physiotherapy we calculated the referral rate per 1000 of the population in each of the individual sites and then by their geographical setting to calculate average national referral rates.

Q What was the average national physiotherapy referral rate found in Scotland?

Please note these rates can only be reliably applied to physiotherapy services in Scotland, although we have no reason to think that they are not more widely applicable; either way, they will help you to consider the issue.

- Overall average referral rate for Scotland 53.5 per 1000.
- Average referral rate for urban settings 44.5 per 1000.
- Average referral rate for semi-rural settings 49 per 1000.
- Average referral rate for rural settings 66 per 1000.

Q Why should there be such a difference?

The type, scope and referral rates of practice differ in all aspects of health-care, including physiotherapy, according to geographical location.

Urban and rural differences

In urban areas, for example, there tends to be a much greater concentration of a range of healthcare providers, both state and privately funded. This means that patients can access many more specialist services, according to their need and preference, more easily. We have found that in terms of physiotherapy, for example, the lower rate of referral experienced in these settings reflected the wider range of providers available.

This is not the case in more rural settings. Patients generally have less choice as there are fewer available providers, hence the increased overall referral rate. By their very nature, healthcare practitioners in more rural settings tend to be more likely to be 'specialist generalists' purely because they have to be.

An experience to learn from

A patient with a specific biomechanical lower-limb problem living in the city of Edinburgh is far more likely to be seen by a specialist podiatrist than if they live more rurally. The same argument can be applied to maternal ante-natal services. Other medical, nursing and allied health professions report similar issues. Healthcare practitioners in more rural settings have to be able to deal with the full range of conditions that come through the door without having the luxury of being able to refer onward as easily and this is reflected in the overall referral rates.

National AHP Census (2005)

In 2005, a one-day census was conducted for the whole of Scotland in an attempt to identify the size and diversity of allied health professionals' case-loads. It was completed by over 80% of qualified allied health professionals in Scotland. Although this exercise did not identify national referral rates by profession, it also identified that the overall rate of referral to therapy services is greater in rural areas. The work focuses on caseloads but has some very interesting results that may be of interest.

A report of this work can be found at www.scotland.gov.uk/publications/2006.

Top tips

- Not sure how to accurately classify populations, practices or areas in terms of geography? Go to Appendix VIII, where we have included the definitions used nationally in Scotland and information about where to find this out for the rest of the UK.
- Look at the range and diversity of conditions your service covers, the more wide-ranging and diverse the more likely it is for your referral rate to be higher than the national norm.
- Use the 'anticipated referral rate calculator' (in Appendix VI) to help you anticipate whether or not you can expect an increase in referral numbers following the introduction of patient self-referral.
- Not sure what the national referral rates are for services similar to yours? Use your professional networks to see if you can make an estimate against which to benchmark yourself. Some information is always better than none.

Waiting lists

The issue of existing waiting lists is frequently brought up as an area of concern by interested parties.

Q What do I do about my waiting list?
Q Can I still introduce self-referral if I have a waiting list? Does it matter?

We are commonly asked these questions. Before we even start to answer, we have to establish some basic facts.

Patient self-referral is not ...

Patient self-referral does not mean the same as immediate access nor should it result in queue-jumping or the introduction of a two-tiered service. You should be very clear in publicising this message from the start to dispel myths and unrealistic expectations among both staff and potential service users.

Again, to expand on this and using the experience within the national physiotherapy self-referral trial, the sites involved had a wide range of waiting times for their services from the outset (0–22 weeks).

What we advocated then still holds true. All effort should be made to reduce your waiting list to an acceptable level before introducing self-referral.

It makes sense to have a manageable system, a waiting time that meets local service standards, staffing complements and other local issues. Having a waiting list does not preclude you from introducing patient self-referral but may make it more difficult to measure its impact.

Consider also that having an excessive waiting list can have a negative impact on the perceptions of those that provide and use these services. If there are few perceived benefits, or any actual benefits, mixed up with the problems directly attributed to excessive waiting lists, it will be so much harder to demonstrate any real benefits or clarify the issues you perceive to be associated with patient self-referral. Without accurate data maintaining support will be much harder.

If you have an excessive waiting list, patients are less likely to bother to refer themselves to your services. This will mean that you will not get a true reflection of the real or true rate of patient self-referral to your service.

Cautionary point

Watch out for the hidden danger of historical under-provision and its effect on waiting lists. Such under-provision, in our experience, results in an increase in the overall referral rate and a possible negative impact on your waiting list.

If you have a service that meets local waiting time standards from the outset, life will be much simpler. We recommend that you make every effort to be in this position. What we do know is that introducing patient self-referral into a system which has longer waiting times will not add anything to the overall service or contribute to reducing waiting times.

Patient self-referral should be seen for what it really is, just another way of widening access to your service, not an additional service implemented to circumvent or deal with waiting times.

Top tips

- Make every effort to reduce any excessive waiting lists before you introduce patient self-referral services.
- It will be well worth the effort and possible time delay this may cause you in the longer term.

Chapter 13

Making critical friends

During the vital planning stage, you need to find out what others think about the concept of introducing patient self-referral. Why? You will need their support throughout but you may have to work at cultivating some of these relationships. This is of particular relevance in systems where services are or can be commissioned, for example current policy in England which encourages primary care trusts and/or practices to commission services on behalf of their populations (also known as 'practice-based commissioning').

What are 'critical friends'?

Critical friends tend to have the following characteristics in common:

- influence
- an interest in innovation
- are focused on improving the patient experience
- meeting organisational objectives
- are fairly senior in the organisation.

Who are your potential 'critical friends'?

Examples of who your potential 'critical friends' could, and should, be include the following:

- patients and their advocacy groups
- board- or senior-level organisational executives and non-executives
- service managers
- business managers
- lead GPs
- individual GP practices
- hospital consultants, in particular those in the specialties for which you provide services
- other major referrers to your service
- public health departments
- local service redesign or improvement leads
- commissioning managers
- funding providers.

You could say that this suggested list should become your family of 'critical friends'.

We do emphasise patients and their role in this. The term 'patient power' was coined for a reason and is at the heart of modern healthcare policy.

Before meeting your 'critical friend' to discuss your ideas you should prepare what amounts to a 'business case' that clearly sets out the following.

- The overall rationale, including political and professional body context.
- The evidence supporting patient self-referral, quoting key sources and the potential benefits for patients and services.
- Facts and figures about your population and service: be specific, include any resource implications you have identified; this is not always doom and gloom, a carefully thought out and presented plan is always well received.
- Projections that not only relate to your service but the potential knock-on effects for others, i.e. potential reduction in investigations, drug prescribing and so on.
- Your Impact Plan (*see* Part III) and your intentions with regard to evaluation and reporting.
- Sources of support gained already.
- The possible relevance and applicability that patient self-referral could have for other services, i.e. you may be making a case for self-referral to your services but will the issues and hence the outcomes may be the same for other services in your organisation? Could your experience inform the development of similar services in the future for other healthcare providers to the benefit of patients and the organisation?

We advocate that, in the first instance, you approach your critical friends more informally.

Top tip

Invite your critical friends around for a cup of coffee to discuss your ideas, but have the facts and figures, forward projections and anticipated benefits – what amounts to your business plan – at your fingertips. Keep patients at the heart of your discussions and let your critical friends know you have done your homework and know what you are talking about!

This less-formal approach in the first instance could be more beneficial over the longer term for several reasons.

- Your critical friends may feel more involved and become advocates for your plans from the outset, increasing your chances of continued support.

- They may have access to other key individuals you may not have thought of or to whom you do not have such ready access.
- You should ask them for their comments on what you have prepared and invite their contributions. They could identify something quite critical that you have overlooked and allow you to modify your ideas.
- Everyone has their own perspective on issues but also targets and objectives to meet. Making their objectives your objectives can not only increase your chance of success but also share the burden during the development stage.
- Presenting a development from a team perspective, especially when it is multi-professional and managerial, is far more powerful than one that just involves one service.

In addition to ensuring that you have a wide circle of critical friends, you also need to ensure that your communication strategy includes other key stakeholders. Key referral sources, GPs for example, will be crucial to your success.

Top tip

Ensure you keep all your stakeholders informed of your emerging plans, in particular the key referring sources. Once your plans are more developed, it might be worthwhile planning on how you can involve these stakeholders.

Top tips

- Know your population and your service. If you don't, make it your business to find out.
- Use the 'referral tool' and 'anticipated referral calculator' to provide you with an indication of potential impact on overall referral numbers.
- Get on top of excessive waiting lists to ensure your waiting time meets local standards.
- Prepare your 'business case'; know your facts.
- Make and maximise the use of critical friends.

Chapter 14

Checklist

You should now complete this checklist before you move on to Part III. If you do not have the answers to any of the elements, make plans to get this information prospectively as it will greatly enhance your chance of success.

Checklist 2

- I know the size of the population my service covers. ☐
- I know what proportion of the population lives in urban, semi-rural or rural areas. ☐
- I know exactly the deprivation indices of each area. ☐
- I know the gender, age and ethnic breakdown of the population and if this differs throughout the area. ☐
- I know if the profile and size of the population has changed over the last three years. ☐
- I know the annual referral rate to my service, expressed as a proportion per 1000 of the population. ☐
- I know the breakdown of referral rates per individual site expressed as a proportion per 1000 of the population. ☐
- I can provide a breakdown of exactly where all these new patients came from, i.e. the exact sources: GPs, consultants, other sources, etc., expressed as a proportion per 1000 of the population. ☐
- I know what investigations or drugs new patients had or were prescribed. ☐
- I know what proportion of referrals is classed as inappropriate. ☐
- I know the exact length of my waiting list and if it has varied over the year. ☐
- I can provide a breakdown of the profile of my patients, i.e. by age, gender, condition, contacts, outcomes, etc. ☐
- I have statistics information about patient employment and/or work absence. ☐
- I know how many patients fail to attend for their first appointment or do not fully complete their course of treatment. ☐
- I know what happens to patients after they are discharged, how many proceed for secondary referral, surgery or other management options. ☐
- I know if my service overlaps with another similar service provider and have agreed how this will be managed. ☐

- I know exactly where my service is provided in terms of whole-time equivalents and sessions. ☐
- I know exactly what my staffing complement is, expressed as whole-time equivalents per grade. ☐
- I know how many students my service accommodates. ☐
- I know what patients think about my service. ☐
- I have made the effort to seek out other services that have developed patient self-referral to ask about their experiences. ☐
- I have made a projection of the anticipated referral rate to my service after introducing self-referral using the tool provided. ☐
- I have made every effort to bring my waiting list into line with locally accepted levels. ☐
- I have reviewed my communications strategy to ensure the formal links within and between my service and other stakeholders, including key referral sources, are functioning adequately. ☐
- I have identified and had a cup of coffee with my family of critical friends to have an informal chat about my plans, although I do not have a clear outline of what the service will entail at this stage. ☐

Chapter 15

Further reading

Association of Chartered Physiotherapy Managers (ACPM) (2001) *Recommendations for Calculating Physiotherapy Staff for GP Referred Musculoskeletal Outpatients*. Chartered Society of Physiotherapy, London.

British Medical Association (2005) *Healthcare in a Rural Setting*. BMA, London (www.bma.org.uk/op.msf/content/healthcarerural/rurality).

Carstairs V and Morris R (1991) *Deprivation and Health in Scotland*. University Press, Aberdeen.

Chartered Society of Physiotherapy (2004) *Making Physiotherapy Count: a range of quality assured services*. CSP, London.

Farmer J, Lauder W, Richards *et al.* (2003) Dr John has gone: assessing health professional contribution to remote rural community sustainability in the UK. *Social Science and Medicine*. **57**: 673–86.

Ferguson A, Griffin E and Mulcahy C (1999) Patient self-referral to physiotherapy in general practice: a model for the new NHS? *Physiotherapy*. **85**: 13–20.

Holdsworth L, Webster V and McFadyen AK (2006) Self-referral to physiotherapy: deprivation and geographical setting: is there a relationship? Results of a national trial. *Physiotherapy*. **92**: 16–25.

Holdsworth L, Webster V and McFadyen A (2006) Are patients who refer themselves to physiotherapy different from those referred by GPs? Results of a national trial. *Physiotherapy*. **92**: 26–33.

Holdsworth L, Webster V and McFadyen A (in press). What are the costs to NHS Scotland of self-referral to physiotherapy? Results of a national trial. *Physiotherapy*.

ISD (2004) *Scottish Health Statistics. Information and Statistics Division, Common Services Agency. Scottish Executive*. HMSO, Edinburgh.

McLoone P (2000) *Carstairs Scores for Scottish Postcode Sectors from the 1991 Census*. Public Health Research Unit, Glasgow.

Scottish Executive (2006) *Allied Health Professionals Count* (www.scotland.gov.uk/publications/2006).

Scottish Executive, Department of Health (2004) *Scottish Executive Urban Rural Classification*. HMSO, Edinburgh.

SIMD (2004) *Scottish Index of Multiple Deprivation*. HMSO, Edinburgh (www.scotland.gov.uk/SIMD2004Data).

Part III

Chapter 16

Preparing for implementation

How will patients refer themselves?

Once you have decided on the type of service you will be introducing, the next step is to work out how patients will actually refer themselves to it.

Whatever you decide, patients will need to provide some basic information about themselves and their condition or problem to assist you in processing their referral efficiently and effectively. At the present time, there are basically two different ways to get this information but we acknowledge that these options may increase as technology advances. It will not be too long until patients are requesting appointments via email, for example, or even by text messaging. Currently, however, the most common ways patients introduce themselves are by telephone or in person.

Telephone

If you opt to receive referrals from patients over the telephone, you will need to think about whether you use the telephone as a means of just receiving referrals or as a patient management tool or as an opportunity for eliciting referrals or information.

The telephone as a referral tool

Patients telephone specifically to ask for an appointment with a healthcare practitioner. They are offered the option to provide details there and then or to be called back for this information at a later time. This could involve a call to a GP surgery, to a healthcare service directly or to a call centre or centralised booking facility.

The telephone as a referral and management tool

Patients telephone a dedicated telephone line where their calls are either logged and they are called back or their calls are responded to by either experienced healthcare practitioners, administration officers or reception personnel. The management of patients can follow a number of pathways, depending on the options available.

- Appointment for further assessment, mutually agreed.
- Patient advised to come to a drop-in clinic, details provided.
- Patient assessed, given advice and discharged from care.

- Patient assessed, given advice, follow-up information sent to the patient's home and discharged from care.
- Patient assessed, given advice, follow-up information sent to the patient's home and patient put on a waiting list to be seen by healthcare practitioner as per waiting list management criteria.
- Patient assessed, given advice, follow-up information sent out to the patient's home and treatment appointment mutually agreed.
- Patient considered not appropriate, referred to GP or other healthcare practitioner.
- Patient assessed considered not appropriate and discharged.
- Patient requires immediate referral to doctor or other healthcare practitioner.

Cautionary point

If the patient is managed completely over the telephone without the need for a face-to-face appointment, how are you going to communicate the result of this consultation to their family doctor or GP?

The telephone as an active elicitor of referrals

We are aware of some services that pro-actively screen all patients who telephone for an appointment with their GP. In this system, all patients are asked by the receptionist if their complaint is something a physiotherapist/ nurse/dietician or so forth might be able to help them with. If the patient states that this might be possible their details are taken and either an appointment with the identified healthcare practitioner is made or arrangements are made for the patient to be contacted at later time.

An experience to learn from

We know of a patient self-referral service in the north-east of England that actively elicits referrals and manages the process very successfully. This service reports referral rates that are approximately 50% higher than similar services that do not actively elicit. This system was introduced gradually but the service had to increase provision to match the rise in referral numbers. The value of such systems lie in the fact that patients are seen by the most appropriate healthcare practitioner more directly in addition to the associated reduction in GP workload.

Points to consider for active eliciting of referrals include the following.

- Eliciting referrals can result in an increase in the number of referrals to your service.

- The time frame in which you handle referrals: this has major implications for services in the UK where there is a government target or standard that all patients requesting an appointment at their GP surgery need to be seen within 48 hours. If patients are diverted to other healthcare services after being 'elicited' this rule still applies. At the time of writing this does not apply in most cases if patients request appointments with healthcare practitioners other than doctors, but you are advised to check this as the rules do differ from region to region and may change in the future.
- There is no point in introducing a system that is known to increase referral rates if you are not sure if you can deal with the patients effectively and efficiently.

Cautionary points

- We strongly recommend that if you are keen to introduce an 'active eliciting' approach, you do this incrementally. Start by using the telephone as a referral tool; only when you are confident in your system should you consider actively eliciting referrals to your service.
- Again, consider how you communicate the result of telephone-only consultations to the patient's doctor.

In person

Using this method, patients present themselves at identified locations and usually refer themselves by completing a form.

Top tips

- Ensure that the system you choose has taken account of the geography and patient profile of your region: there is no reason for not having a combination of systems running in parallel.
- Patients may value an opportunity to telephone to arrange an appointment/call back/to access triage/advice, particularly if they live more remotely or have mobility problems.
- Check to see if national or local waiting time standards apply to your service.
- Only consider introducing active eliciting systems once you are confident in your overall ability to meet potential demand.
- Ensure you have considered how the results of your patient contact is communicated with the patient's doctor.

Chapter 17

Publicising the change in access to your service

By now you should have a good idea about what kind of service you are planning to introduce. It is time therefore to consider how you will inform its potential users and other key stakeholders of these changes.

Q How do I go about telling patients and other staff?

There is no point in introducing changes to services that rely on patients referring themselves if they do not know they can actually do this. It will therefore be necessary for you to develop a publicity or marketing strategy.

The approach you adopt will depend on whether or not you will be offering patient self-referral to the full population you serve or just an element of it.

Full population access

If you intend to offer self-referral to all patients within your local population you have many more options available. You can adopt a much wider marketing campaign which could include all or a blend of the following.

Posters

- Ensure you involve service users in poster development – do not assume you can decide that they will understand your message. Ask them!
- Design posters detailing the service.
- Do not try to put every piece of information about 'what you do' on a poster.
- Specify how your service can be accessed.
- Guide potential referrers to more detailed information, i.e. pick up a leaflet at your library, community centre, GP surgery, etc.
- Include some key information as to what type of conditions would be appropriate for your service.

- Specify what kind of service you are providing, for example if you have drop-in clinics or a telephone advice service.
- Include opening times and location of clinics.
- How patients can refer themselves.
- If you have referral forms for patients to complete where can they be accessed?
- Where will the posters be displayed, for example health clinics, local library, clubs, community centres, etc.
- Enlist the help of a local information technologist or marketing person to ensure your posters are more likely to be noticed.
- Ensure you have resources to continue to update and replace your posters as and when required.
- Ensure language and format requirements have been addressed.

Top tips

- Keep your poster focused, accurate and eye-catching.
- Direct your potential referrers to other sources of additional information, i.e. leaflets, web addresses, etc.

Leaflets

- Ensure you involve service users in their design – do not assume that they will understand your message. Ask them!
- Produce clear simple leaflets which contain the same information as detailed above in the poster section.
- Include clear information that tells patients how to refer themselves.
- Ensure language and format requirements are addressed.

Presentations

- The presentations you may have made to your staff and critical friends can be used when explaining the service to other healthcare professionals.
- Presentations can be delivered to user groups, community groups and local volunteers. Remember to ensure that the language you use in these types of presentations does not include technical or jargonised terms or abbreviations: 'plain English' is needed here.

Q Where should I display posters and leaflets?

This will depend on the population you wish to reach but you can consider any or all of the following:

- GP practices
- health clinics
- therapy departments
- accident and emergency departments
- community centres
- libraries
- leisure centres
- local shops.

You can also target specific groups, for example:

- senior citizen groups
- mother and toddler groups
- sports groups
- local condition specific voluntary groups, i.e. the Arthritis and Musculo-skeletal Alliance (ARMA).

Top tip

Don't forget to let other healthcare staff know about your service: word of mouth is still one of the most powerful publicity tools there is!

An experience to learn from

One community advertised its patient self-referral service in local pubs, hotels and restaurants as well as the range of places identified above – and was surprisingly successful!

Media features

- Consider placing a feature in the local staff publication.
- Local press may run a feature in the home and health or local news section.
- Local radio, including hospital radio, will reach different audiences.

The world wide web

Where do patients find out about which private therapy healthcare practitioners there are in their area? Two of the most popular ways used these are to look up services:

- in the telephone directory
- on the internet.

NHS services have not been so creative about publicising their services to the public. Try 'googling' your profession, i.e. 'occupational therapy' or 'physiotherapy' with 'NHS services' and your local area, and see what comes up. The likelihood is that the answer will not be a lot!

Top tip

Speak to your local friendly information technologist or communications staff again. Can anything be done to publicise your service on the world wide web?

Limited population access

If you are introducing patient self-referral to just a sub-section of your population, you will have to ensure that you tailor your publicity accordingly to avoid confusion and possible inappropriate self-referral. This may require targeting patients directly via newsletters, leaflets or personal approaches.

You might expect that the amount of publicity you generate should correlate directly with the uptake of service but the experience in other countries tells us otherwise. Even with blanket publicity, using all the methods above, the self-referral rate still remains at under 30% of all referrals as experienced in New South Wales, Australia and an even lower rate in Florida, USA. From our own work some of the locations reported that they felt they had to keep raising awareness of self-referral as their rate dropped after the first flourish of publicity died down.

Changing patterns of behaviour, in particular longstanding ones, does not happen overnight. It will be some time before members of the UK public automatically think they can refer themselves to a range to healthcare services in the same way they currently do for dentistry.

Top tips

- Seek the involvement of user groups, community groups and members of the public when developing your publicity strategy – it should appeal to, and be clearly understood by, your intended population. Remember cultural differences may make your message inaccessible. Seek guidance on adapting parts of your strategy.
- Target your intended population appropriately.
- Don't forget to inform other healthcare providers.
- Think creatively about where you place your publicity material and renew it regularly.
- Think big, think the www!

Chapter 18

Measuring and demonstrating impact

The importance of being able to demonstrate impact cannot be over-emphasised. It needs to be carefully considered and pro-actively planned from the outset. Doing this well will rely on the approach you take to measuring, what and how you measure and the reliability of your data.

Most frequently asked questions

Q How do I go about measuring the impact of introducing patient self-referral?

Q What data should I be using?

Q How do I collect this?

Q What should I do with this information once I've got it?

Why information is needed

To survive in today's healthcare delivery sector, services need to be able to demonstrate their clinical and cost effectiveness on an ongoing basis. This is particularly so for newly introduced or redesigned services. Not only is this a professional requirement, it is also needed to provide assurance that standards of care are being met, that there are positive benefits for patients and services, and that value for money is demonstrated. A rolling programme of impact planning, guideline implementation, clinical audit and patient and staff feedback should be integral to service delivery.

Traditionally, demonstrating impact has not been a strong point for most services. Consistently, we have struggled with demonstrating what impact, if any, we make on patient care and in delivering healthcare policies. This means that, in an environment where there is ever-increasing competition for scarce resources, an inability to make a credible case severely hampers any ability to attract ongoing or additional support.

Major effort needs to be put into planning how the impact of introducing patient self-referral will be demonstrated. You need this to be able to demonstrate the impact on patients, on your service, on referral sources and other services, and how it meets organisational and national objectives.

How do you measure impact?

In order to demonstrate impact, you need to know what to measure. Some things are obvious, for example how many patients self-referred compared to those referred from other sources and also in comparison with baseline data. Other measures of impact are more complex or subtle but may prove to be very useful to you in the future. This is why you need to put considerable thought into this from the outset and have an 'impact plan'.

Top tip

All organisations have objectives that tend to be developed and reviewed regularly based on a combination of national, professional and local issues. You need to be fully aware of what these are. If in doubt, there are a number of key people in any organisation who should be able to update you and provide the necessary information. These can include clinical directors, performance, business and organisational managers.

Formulating your impact plan

Having an impact plan provides you with a unique opportunity to bring together all the objectives of your organisation, service and profession. Normally, these tend to be separate documents. Bringing them together allows you to look at the overall picture and helps to ensure that you have considered all perspectives and will be able to provide reliable information. It allows you to identify the key objectives that are directly relevant to your service generally and patient self-referral specifically.

Formulating an impact plan may sound complicated, but if you follow the steps below, it should be relatively straightforward.

- Start by drawing up a table with two columns.
- Compile a list in the left-hand column that includes the key objectives of your organisation, which should include a combination of:
  - national
  - clinical
  - organisational
  - human resource issues.

- Add key:
  - professional or national organisational guidelines or standards
  - any other issues that you consider should be included that may be relevant to your service; what about community issues?
- Think widely at this stage.

Table 18.1 has been compiled for demonstration purposes only and contains a sample range of objectives that a physiotherapy service may identify as appropriate for further consideration when demonstrating the impact of patient self-referral.

Table 18.1 Samples of objectives when demonstrating the impact of patient self-referral

Objective	Data needed as evidence
Provide primary healthcare practitioner appointments within 48 hours of request	
Decrease inappropriate referrals to specialist services	
Achieve 3% saving on drugs	
Ensure that patients are offered access to appropriate services close to home	
Patients are involved in the planning and evaluation of services	
Patients are assessed in line with professionally determined standards	
Patients are provided with appropriate information	
Improve patient outcomes	
Demonstrate high levels of patient satisfaction with healthcare provision	
All staff members have a personal development plan (PDP)	
Minimise absence from paid employment	

When compiling this list, explore all sources of information, including the web-based information about your organisation for clues. Do not forget to think laterally and prospectively; for example, if one of the organisational objectives relates to waiting times for what are currently predominantly medical specialties, think about how introducing patient self-referral to existing and extended roles could improve matters; this may not have been factored in, or, if there are objectives relating to the prescribing of drugs or specialist investigations, think about how self-referral could potentially offer a more cost and clinically effective alternative.

Once you have your list of relevant objectives, in the right-hand column of the table start to list the key data items you will need to provide evidence that you are meeting or impacting on the objective.

This information should include patient demographic, clinical and staff-related data; the key things you need to provide you with an overview of how the service is functioning (*see* Table 18.2). Think widely, do you want to know your re-referral rate or the investigations your patients have?

Table 18.2 Samples of objectives when demonstrating the impact of patient self-referral*

Objective	Data needed as evidence
Provide primary healthcare practitioner appointments within 48 hours of request	Date of referral and when assessed
Decrease inappropriate referrals to specialist services	Secondary referral rates
Achieve 3% saving on drugs	Prescribing details by referral source
Ensure that patients are offered access to appropriate services close to home	Location details – proportional breakdown
Patients are involved in the planning and evaluation of services	Patient involvement and feedback details
Patients are assessed in line with professionally determined standards	Service standards
Patients are provided with appropriate information	Audit of information strategy and patient feedback
Improve patient outcomes	Outcome measures from clinicians, staff and patient perspectives
Demonstrate high levels of patient satisfaction with healthcare provision	Patient experience information
All staff members have a personal development plan (PDP)	PDP audit
Minimise patient and staff absence from paid employment	Employment and absence details

* This is just a sample and not an exhaustive list.

Table 18.2 constitutes your impact plan. It should clearly identify what types of data or information you need to collect to demonstrate the impact of your service and how it is contributing to meeting key objectives.

> Top tips
>
> - Develop an impact plan.
> - Link self-referral to key organisation and service objectives.
> - Think laterally, be creative.
> - Review and update regularly.
> - Exploit the expertise of others, including your critical friends.

What information should you collect?

Realistically, once you have compiled your impact plan you will probably realise that you are already collecting much of the data needed. It may be that you just need to review the overall dataset and update it slightly it in light of your impact plan.

What is crucial though is that you have a good understanding of the existing service before you start to introduce patient self-referral. Ensure you have reliable baseline data as outlined earlier in Part II.

> Top tips
>
> - If you don't have this data, as we advised before, it is in your interest to collate some information before introducing the new service even if it is just a reflection of the last three months. We are aware of services that have not done this and were therefore unable to demonstrate the impact patient self-referral had had in a credible and robust way.
> - If you do have baseline data, how confident are you in its accuracy? It may be worth undertaking a small-scale validation exercise to be really sure.

An experience to learn from

A service we know was convinced that it had reliable information about the number of the referrals it received by source. The service used a well-known computer system to register and follow patient contacts. It came to light that the data they were providing to the study centre did not match what their computer system reported. After extensive scrutiny of the information technology service, a major problem was found in the coding system of the computer and the service had, in fact, been using completely invalid data for the last five years! This would never have come to light if the 'mismatch' had not alerted them – always better to undertake a small validation study to be sure and repeat it from time to time.

Top tip

Don't fall into the trap of just collecting data about the new service or just about self-referrals. To make meaningful comparisons and demonstrate impact, not only do you need good baseline data, but information on *all* referrals to your service.

Self-referral dataset

The next stage will be to have an agreed dataset that will allow you to collect all the data needed for ongoing monitoring of your service and to demonstrate the impact of introducing patient self-referral.

Top tip

Only collect what you really need!

A copy of the dataset that was used in the national physiotherapy trial undertaken in Scotland during 2003–2005 can be found in Appendix III. Although it was developed primarily for physiotherapy use, we are confident that over 90% of the data items are relevant to all services. Profession-related modifications may be needed to some of the definitions that accompany the data set, however. If you wish to use it, we recommend that it is reviewed and cross-referenced against your impact plan to ensure that it meets your local needs. We also include in Appendix IV a copy of information developed as part of the Chartered Society of Physiotherapy Sharing Effective Practice Project (SEPP) to inform this process. Again, this has multi-professional relevance.

National Trial Self-referral Dataset

This contains the ability to record: demographic, referral and clinical elements; patient and physiotherapy intervention outcomes; employment and work absence; previous service use; investigations, drugs and onward referrals.

Defining the dataset

How data are defined, that is, how they are interpreted and applied in practice will dictate how reliable and useful information will be. Staff using the dataset must be fully aware of which definitions to use and apply them consistently. You must ensure that as much subjectivity as possible is eliminated from the start.

Top tip

It is worthwhile spending time with staff both individually and in teams to make sure they are confident, are applying terms consistently and know what is expected of them. Let them get used to using the dataset and offer feedback sessions to reinforce issues and address concerns. Go through the full dataset with staff ensuring that they are consistently applying the definitions. Do not 'go live' until you are confident that staff members are comfortable and proficient in applying the definitions and using the dataset. You will be doomed if you rush this!

A copy of the definitions that accompany the national dataset can be accessed by visiting www.selfreferralphysioinfo.com. You need to ensure you have accurate definitions for aspects of the data set you decide to use.

An experience to learn from

We sometimes think that the way we define something is universally used by our colleagues in the healthcare setting. This is not always the case. An example of this comes from a speech and language therapy service which became aware that its staff members were not applying the same definitions for patient discharge reasons. Some staff members were recording patients who were discharged after failing to attend for their first appointment under the category of 'Patient failed to complete their course of treatment' whilst other staff members categorised them as 'Patient failed to attend for first appointment'. This may seem pedantic but it was very important to this service to be able to capture this information accurately.

> **Top tips**
>
> - Have or obtain accurate baseline data.
> - Have an agreed dataset and definitions that can deliver your impact plan.
> - As far as possible, use validated and standardised definitions and scales.
> - Ensure that all staff members are proficient and signed up to the service.
> - Be prepared to pilot the dataset.

Collecting data

Once you have your agreed data definitions and dataset, you need to think about how data will be collected in practice. Most likely, clinical staff will be using a paper-based system that will involve providing the required data to a central point via a pre-printed form. It should be recognised, however, that some services, although admittedly still in the minority, are 'paperless', with clinical staff directly inputting patient-related data at the 'patientside'. Whichever method suits your situation, we advise that you consider the following.

- Try to avoid introducing another set of paperwork to meet your new information demands. You may find it more productive to review your total approach to patient record-keeping to make life easier for staff members; you are also more likely to receive accurate data in this way. There are a number of options available to you. Having pre-printed carbonised sheets that double up as the definitive patient record as well as data-inputting sheets is a possibility. Speak to your medical records department and/or data protection officer to ensure that whatever method you introduce complies with current legislation.
- Try to keep your data requirements to a maximum of one A4 sheet.
- Make as many data items as possible into simple tick boxes, minimising the need for free and ambiguous text.
- Think about how you get the data sheets from the 'patientside' to the computer. Is this a manual or postal exercise? Is this a daily or weekly requirement? By how long after discharge do you need the sheets to be input?
- Ensure that any computerised record system contains your key data requirements and can be collated easily. Spend time discussing with your IT support what data you need to be collated and how you want to express it. Taking time to consider and set up appropriate 'reports' at this stage will make your data collection appropriate and streamlined.

> **Top tips**
>
> - Only collect what you need.
> - Minimise duplication: try to have a single approach that meets data-collection and record-keeping purposes.
> - Make the process straightforward, logical and unambiguous.
> - Consider timescales and set clear standards so that staff members know what is expected.
> - Provide regular service and individual feedback.

How should you process the data?

The ways in which service data can be processed are numerous. We don't intend to provide any in-depth advice as to the options available, which range from basic paper-based systems to stand-alone, hand-held, networked or web-based electronic systems. By far the most resource-efficient and, if planned properly, robust method is by using an electronic or computer-based system. These days most services have access to some sort of electronic system that has either been bought 'off the shelf' or developed in-house by a helpful information technologist.

> **Top tips**
>
> - It is always useful to write a list of the key information or reports you will need to extract from your data *before* you implement the new dataset. This is your opportunity to put down on paper many of the questions you have asked yourself about your service in the past but have possibly never had the data to answer reliably. Compile your list using your impact plan cross-referenced with your dataset. Include items that are not just straightforward reports, for example you may need to know the numbers of referrals to your service for a given time, but you may also want a breakdown by source of referral, age and gender or whether patients who failed to complete their course of treatment have a particular condition or come from a particular referral source.
> - Once you have your list, ensure that your system can answer these queries. If it cannot, it may be quite simple to rectify but require the input of your friendly information technologist once again. This is your opportunity to really get to the bottom of your service information needs, providing benefits wider than just the patient self-referral elements.

Using your information for maximum impact

As the saying goes, 'information is knowledge and knowledge is power'. If you have gone to all the trouble of determining what your information needs are and how you are going to get them, you need to use this information to maximum effect.

Basically, there are two reasons for you to have accurate information about your service:

- to monitor progress for your own use
- to report impact to others.

Monitoring

You will need to monitor your service to ensure that it is meeting its objectives and to identify trends and where modifications may have to be factored in. Monitoring is a key aspect of managing your service effectively. This is particularly so in the initial stages and much of the information you monitor will be for your use only.

Top tips

- Identify what you need to monitor and when.
- Refer back to your impact plan.
- Ensure you are involving the views of service users and providers.

Engaging service users and providers

Irrespective of how well you have planned your service, if it doesn't meet the perceived or actual needs of its users, it will not succeed. We recommend that you involve service users from the earliest stages of your development. Invite representatives to sit on your steering or development group.

Not only do you have to elicit users' views but you should have identified mechanisms for providing feedback to them so they know their views are both valued and acted on. One way of doing this is to develop a user newsletter that can distributed to new service users to encourage their involvement. Consider setting up a users' group as part of ongoing service monitoring.

Feedback from staff is equally important, particularly in the early stages. Make it very clear that you expect and value their input at all stages in the development, delivery and evaluation of the service. Staff members, along with patients, will be your greatest ambassadors.

> **Top tips**
>
> - Actively include service users in your development plans from the outset.
> - Follow up service users to capture their views.
> - Staff providing the service should also be similarly engaged.
> - Act on your findings.
> - Provide feedback to both users and staff.

A sample of service user and staff questionnaires used in physiotherapy self-referral services can be found on the internet by visiting www. selfreferralphysioinfo.com.

Reporting impact results

Who should you be reporting to? Who is your audience?

For exactly the same reasons as outlined in Chapter 13, 'Making critical friends', whom you choose to tell about the impact of your patient self-referral service is also very important. Don't underestimate how powerful this can be.

There can be significant benefits for a service if it can engage with a wide range of stakeholders, including patients. The more benefits the better, as some stakeholders may not have previously appreciated the contribution your service can make to their overall agendas. Demonstrate the impact of your service in terms that are particularly relevant to the intended audience. Remember, we previously advised you to make their objectives your objectives. Providing a report that meets this purpose will be very well-received.

It will be in your interest to really put some thought into determining who needs to be told about the impact of your service. Not exhaustive by any means, but the list could include:

- patients, in the widest sense, from individuals to advocacy groups, voluntary organisations, local health councils and so forth
- the clinical team
- other clinical teams which may be interested in patient self-referral
- business managers
- service managers
- medical and nursing directors
- directors of public health
- chief executive officers
- community service managers

- service commissioners, including insurance companies if appropriate
- relevant professional bodies or networks.

Top tips

- In addition to specifically targeting information at individuals or teams, consider also adopting a more general dissemination approach. Does your organisation have an annual report, newsletter or other means of communicating with staff, patients, other agencies and the wider public? We would also recommend that you start to explore the implications of publishing your impact report via the www to widen dissemination. Speak to your information technologist once again.
- Let your professional organisation know of any areas of good practice or issues you feel should be shared widely.

What should you be reporting?

The content of your report should vary according to the intended audience. This principle also applies to the frequency of reports. Be prepared to make reports on an interim basis as required but to your staff in particular so they are kept up to date.

For example, the chief executive of your organisation may be primarily concerned with demonstrating to the higher echelons the extent to which the organisation is achieving the government's set targets. This may mean that you will need to emphasise the impact of your service on waiting times, efficiency of resource usage and access, for example.

Other audiences, patient representative groups for example, may also be concerned with these matters as well as others taken from their perspective so include outcomes that are tangible to them as well, for example convenience, decreased work absence, patient choice and experience.

Keep the focus on patients as service users

Irrespective of your intended audience, ensure that you include patient-centred impact measures, and don't forget to include their views of the service – now more commonly called the 'patient voice'. It can be incredibly powerful.

Although, and quite understandably, you will wish to highlight the positively reported experiences, it can also be very helpful to identify aspects that were not so well-received so long as you demonstrate that you have listened to these concerns and addressed them or have plans to do so.

An experience to learn from

A service received feedback from patients that although they were delighted with being able to refer themselves and the care they had received; they were not so happy with having to travel across the town to access the service. The service used this information together with other key outcome measurements, i.e. waiting time improvements, patient outcomes, less reliance on other healthcare services, to lobby for resources to secure a further location for this service on the right side of town.

Top tips

- Tailor your report to the intended audience. Be prepared to produce various versions. Don't just circulate one report to all stakeholders if you want to achieve maximum and meaningful impact.
- Use your critical friends again. Ask them for their feedback on what you have written before it is circulated formally.
- Include the patient voice.
- Think about the most appropriate style and format of presentation.
- Be creative!

Reporting format choices

There are more ways of presenting your results than just in a traditional report format. Consider your options. Remember the primary purpose of producing a report is to convey key results and messages. If you haven't grabbed the reader's attention within the first 30 seconds then it won't be read!

Top tips

- A more informal newsletter style may be more appropriate for a range of audiences, including staff, service users and the wider public.
- There is no reason why you cannot use other interesting media: video, CD and so on, for disseminating and demonstrating the impact of your service.
- If you do adopt a traditional report style, remember to preface it with a one-page executive summary. This should be pithy and punchy

and encapsulate the key findings drawing the reader in to read the full report.

- Some of the most powerful messages are the shortest ones!

Top five tips

- Monitor your service closely.
- Include the patient voice.
- Know whom you should be communicating with and that it is relevant to their agenda.
- Make the most of every opportunity to widen your network of critical friends and supporters.
- Think out of the box: use communication options creatively and share your experiences widely.

Chapter 19

Checklist

You should now complete this checklist before you move to Part IV. Missing elements may severely compromise your ability to successfully implement and demonstrate the impact of your patient self-referral service.

Checklist 3

- I am clear about what kind of patient self-referral service best meets the needs of my population, the local geography and the capabilities of my service. ☐
- I am clear what the service will be called, and I will use this title consistently at all times. ☐
- I have worked out how patients will refer themselves to the service. ☐
- I have a publicity strategy. ☐
- I have identified all organisational, clinical and service key objectives that are relevant to my service. ☐
- I have produced an impact plan. ☐
- I have developed an agreed dataset. ☐
- I have definitions for all data. ☐
- I have verified staff understanding of data and data definitions. ☐
- I have decided on a system for collecting and processing the data, that is, paper, computer. ☐
- I have included all the above in my updated business plan. ☐
- I have shared my business plan with my critical friends. ☐
- I have reviewed my communications strategy to ensure that the formal links within and between my service and other stakeholders, including key referral sources, are functioning adequately. ☐
- I know what and when I need to monitor. ☐
- I know my intended audiences. ☐
- I will tailor the key elements of reports or presentations according to audience. ☐
- I have thought about the most appropriate format for reporting my results according to audience. ☐

Chapter 20

Further reading

Avis M, Bond M and Arthur A (1995) Satisfying solutions? A review of some unresolved issues in measuring patient satisfaction. *Journal of Advanced Nursing*. **22**: 316–22.

Crout K, Tweedie JH and Miller DJ (1998) Physical therapists opinions and practices regarding direct access. *Physical Therapy*. **78**: 52–61.

Fulop N, Allen P, Clarke A *et al*. (eds) (2002) *Studying the Organisation and Delivery of Health Services: research methods*. Routledge, London.

McIver S and Meredith P (1998) Patient surveys. There for the asking. *Health Service Journal*. **108**: 26–7.

Mitchell JM and de Lissovoy G (1997) A comparison of resources use and cost in direct access versus physician referral episodes of physical therapy. *Physical Therapy*. **77**: 10–18.

Sheppard L (1994) Public perception of physiotherapy: implications for marketing. *Australian Journal of Physiotherapy*. **40**: 265–71.

Sitzia J and Wood N (1997) Patient satisfaction: a review of issues and concepts. *Social Science and Medicine*. **45**: 1829–43.

Wilcock PM, Brown GCS, Bateson J *et al*. (2003) Inspire quality improvement within the NHS Modernisation Agency collaborative programmes. *Journal of Clinical Nursing*. **12**: 422–30.

Williams KS, Assassa RP, Smith NKG *et al*. (2000) Development, implementation and evaluation of a nurse led continence service: a pilot study. *Journal of Nursing*. **9**: 566–73.

Wilkinson JR and Murray SA (1998) Assessment in primary care: practical issues and possible approaches. *BMJ*. **316**: 1524–8.

Part IV

Chapter 21

Final countdown to implementation

You are now ready to think about introducing your patient self-referral service. You should have:

- done your homework
- gained the support of your critical friends and organisation
- developed your plans for your patient self-referral service.

You now need to think about timescales, about when you plan to introduce the service.

Testing your new system

However thorough your preparation, we still recommend that you test your new service over a three-month 'run-in' period. This was the time needed by the 30 locations at which we introduced patient self-referral to iron out and rectify any chinks in their systems. It was also the time it took for publicity strategies to have an impact. Think of this time as an opportunity to be reassured yourself and to reassure others that you are thoroughly prepared.

> Q Is there a better time of year to introduce a self-referral service?

We have been asked this question on more than occasion, and the simple answer is 'No'. Our advice has remained the same. The introduction does need to be thoughtfully planned but is more influenced by the local situation. If you know that for the next two months or so you will be unusually short-staffed because of leave, for example, you may wish to postpone the introduction of the service until your staffing complement is healthier.

Alternatively, if you know that you are coming into a usually quiet time in terms of referral numbers – major holiday periods, for example – this may prove the ideal opportunity to give staff a little extra time to get to grips with the new procedures.

Be prepared to monitor and review all aspects of the new service over the run-in period at regular intervals. Examine the data collected, engage with staff and service users to find out their views, and ensure that you involve them in your feedback at all stages.

Chapter 22

Publicising the launch of your service

There is no point in advertising your service to the public and potential service users until you are actually ready to receive self-referrals. This will only cause confusion and frustration in the system.

Top tips

Launch your publicity strategy at the same time as you embark on the three-month run-in period. Although the response may be slow to start with, it will allow you the opportunity to ensure that:

- your publicity strategy is reaching your audience
- your referral mechanisms are rigorous and efficient
- your staff are prepared and confident in all aspects of the system's administration
- your approach to data collection and definition are appropriate and unambiguous
- you can monitor and potentially report on the impact accurately.

Cautionary point

Do not think that the number of patients self-referring during the run-in period is indicative of future demand. It takes a long time for the wider public to become aware of changes to systems of healthcare and also to have the confidence to use them.

Be prepared to modify your approach or tools before you formally launch the service.

Chapter 23

The final countdown

Do not proceed until you can confidently say the following.

- I have completed checklists 1, 2 and 3 (and this one!). ☐
- My waiting list meets local standards. ☐
- I have factored in my three-month run-in period. ☐
- My staff are well prepared and signed up. ☐
- I have made my plans for monitoring and evaluation. ☐
- I know how I am going to engage service users and service providers. ☐
- I have a firm date for review. ☐
- I have communicated my plans to key stakeholders, including referral sources, staff and patient groups. ☐

Done all that? Then now you are ready to go! And good luck.

Sample referral forms

NHS Logo here

> **XXXX Health Centre: Patient Self-Referral**
> **Physiotherapy Request Form**

Please complete the following information about yourself and then hand it in to the receptionist. The physiotherapist will contact you to arrange a convenient time for your appointment. Please make sure that you give details as to how you can be most easily contacted to arrange your appointment. If, for whatever reason, you find that you do no longer require a physiotherapy appointment, then please ring the medical centre and leave a message for the physiotherapist.

Today's date: _____   Your date of birth: _____

Name: _____

Address: _____   Daytime phone no. _____

               _____   Other number: _____

Postcode   _____   GP name   _____

Please give a **brief** description of why you want a physiotherapy appointment giving details of what kind of problem you have, how long you have had your problem and how badly its affecting you. Please also provide details if you are experiencing any recent numbness, tingling or muscle weakness.

Have you consulted you GP about this problem?   **YES**   **NO**

Once completed, hand or send this form back to the medical centre.
If you find that your symptoms get worse while you wait to see the physiotherapist then you are advised to see you GP.

NHS Logo here

Self-Referral to Physiotherapy – Name of Town

Please complete this form to refer yourself to physiotherapy and return it to the
Health Centre reception desk

Name: _____   GP name: _____

Address: _____   Date of birth   _/_/_

_____   Date of referral   _/_/_

Phone number (home)_____

(work) _____

Presenting complaint and brief description of symptoms, ie back pain/knee pain:

How long have you had this complaint?

Days ☐   Weeks ☐   Months ☐   Years☐

Is the problem:

New ☐   Exacerbation of old ☐   Ongoing ☐

Have you had this problem before?

Yes ☐   No ☐

(please give details)

Has this problem previously been treated with physiotherapy?

Yes ☐   No ☐

Are the symptoms worsening?

Yes ☐   No ☐

(if yes please give details)

Are you off work/unable to care for a dependant because of this problem?

Yes ☐   No ☐   Not applicable ☐

Using a scale of 0 to 10, score your average level of pain, where 0 is no pain and 10 is the worst
possible pain

    0   1   2   3   4   5   6   7   8   9   10

Please give details of any other treatment you have received for these symptoms:

If you have back and leg pain, have you developed problems with your bladder or bowel?

Yes ☐   No ☐

---

*If at all your symptoms worsen before you receive a physiotherapy appointment, you
are advised to see your GP*

*We will contact you within 2 weeks on the phone number provided above to arrange
a convenient appointment. Please double check to ensure we have the correct
number*

Sample poster

SELF REFERRAL TO PHYSIOTHERAPY

We have changed the way that you can get an appointment to see the physiotherapist here in town name

This means that you do NOT have to visit your GP first

If you feel that you could benefit from seeing the physiotherapist, ask at reception for more details

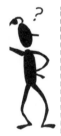

Not sure if physiotherapy is right for you?

Physiotherapy can be particularly beneficial if you are suffering from any of the following:

Low back pain
Neck pain
Recent injuries – *strains and sprains*
Joint and Muscular pain

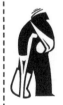

Other conditions are also appropriate for physiotherapy – ask at the health centre reception for further information if you're unsure

Remember, if you suffer an injury, the physiotherapist can advise you on how to manage your injury best - the sooner you see the physiotherapist, the sooner you'll recover

National self-referral dataset

The data definitions that accompany this dataset can be found at www.selfreferralphysioinfo.com.

Patient Self Referral to Physiotherapy – Sample Data Sheet

Patient Name--   Patient Postcode ----------------------

Date of 1st GP consult (GP refs ONLY) ____/____/____   Referral Date ____/____/____

Initial Ass Date ____/____/____   Pat. Gender Male ☐   Female ☐   Date of Birth ____/____/____

Referral Type   Self ☐ GP ☐   GP suggested ☐   Other(Please state)------------------------

Duration of Symptoms   < =2 weeks ☐   2-6 weeks ☐   7-12 weeks ☐   >12 weeks ☐

Employment Status   Paid Employment ☐   Student ☐   Retired ☐

House person ☐   Unemployed ☐

If in paid employment, total No. of days off work as a   ☐☐☐   days
consequence of this condition (*put in 000 if not applicable*)

Condition Category: LBP ☐   Neck ☐   Thoracic ☐   Knee ☐   LL ☐ Multi ☐

UL ☐   Shld ☐   Neuro ☐   Urolog ☐   Other ☐   (Please state)......................

Previous Physio. Y   N   No. Referrals ☐☐   Severity Mild ☐ Moderate ☐   Severe ☐

Subjective Severity of Condition-
Patients Initial Score 0 –100 (0 = no symptoms, 100 = worst symptoms)   ☐☐☐

Discharge Date ____/____/____   Total No. of contacts ☐☐

Discharge reason: Rx Completed ☐   Failed to Complete ☐   Condition resolved 1st appoint ☐

Re-referred to GP (why?)_____   Other _____

Outcome: Goals not recorded ☐   Goals not achieved ☐   Partially Achieved ☐

Achieved (longer than anticipated) ☐   Achieved ☐   Achieved (quicker than anticipated) ☐

Patient Final Subjective Score   0 –100 (0 = no symptoms, 100 = worst possible symptoms)   ☐☐☐

Was the patient prescribed any of the following by their GP before or during this Physiotherapy
intervention ?   YES   NO
        NSAIDs   ☐   ☐
        Painkillers   ☐   ☐   Other (Please state) ————————————

Did the patient undergo any of the following related to this condition up to 3 months prior to or during
the physiotherapy episode of care
X-Ray ☐   MRI Scan ☐   Referral to Secondary Care ☐
                  Other Investigation (Please state) _____

Additional comments can be made on the reverse of this sheet

Sharing effective physiotherapy practice (SEPP) dataset

This work was originally published within the Chartered Society of Physiotherapy publication, *Sharing Effective Physiotherapy Practice* (CSP, 2004). The table contained suggestions for physiotherapists about what sort of information outpatient services should consider collecting. Although developed for physiotherapy use, it is also highly relevant to any service provider as the issues are just the same.

Overview

Reproduced with the kind permission of the Chartered Society of Physio-therapy, London.

You might wish to consider collecting the following information when planning / introducing an out-patient musculoskeletal service. It is acknowledged that in addition, there may be other local or national information you may also want to collect. This information however, provides a comprehensive dataset that will help you to build an evidence base for the service and provide the means to thoroughly describe its rationale *(why?)* and make-up *(how?)*, the impact it has made and the outcomes achieved (*so what?*). It will also allow you to examine the cost effectiveness of the service and provide meaningful comparisons to support future developments.

General Information
- Description of the population the service area covers i.e. size, urban/rural, deprivation
- Prevalence rates among the general population
- How the clinical condition / service area features in national or local health plans / strategies
- The evidence base including any professional or organisational standards relating to this condition i.e. CSP, NICE, SIGN

Service Information
If developing a completely new service, you should ensure that you have baseline information that relates to the year BEFORE the service was introduced to allow comparison and evaluation.

Baseline Data
- Number of referrals made to orthopaedic services per annum by type i.e. spinal, peripheral joint, knee etc (include diagnostic codes if possible)
- Waiting times
- Source of referrals i.e. GP Open access, other sources
- Where the service is provided, i.e. location
- Who provides the service i.e. number and profession / grade of staff (WTE)
- Gender and Age breakdown (use nationally defined age groups)
- Proportion of out-patient referrals that proceed to physiotherapy
- Proportion of out-patient referrals that proceed to surgery
- Re-referral rate

Developing the Service
- Training requirements for staff
- Competencies required including description of scope of practice i.e. level of experience, injection therapy, acupuncture, ability to order investigations, prescribing etc
- Referral and management guidelines / pathways developed
- Patient involvement in development process
- Patient Information
- Communication strategies with referrers and other key staff and patient groups
- Where the service is provided, i.e. location
- Who provides the service i.e. number and profession / grade of staff (WTE)
- Time/s of day when the service operates

Provide timescales for periods described. It is more usual to report figures based on yearly activity.

Service Description
- Waiting times
- Number of referrals made to service
- Number of referrals made to orthopaedic services per annum by type i.e. spinal, peripheral joint, knee etc include diagnostic codes if possible)
- Source of referrals i.e. GP Open access, other sources?
- DNA at first appointment rate
- Gender and Age breakdown (use nationally defined age groups)
- Appropriateness of referral based on defined criteria
- Employment status & work absence
- Assessment tools used (validated?) include a measure of the patients perception of the severity of their problem
- Investigations undertaken including X-rays, scans, blood tests etc
- Management plan including type/s of intervention & information provided
- Number of total service contacts
- Discharge reason i.e. re-referred, intervention complete, failed to complete etc

Outcomes
Use validated scales, if at all possible, if not, provide a reason. Record:
- A measure of outcome of intervention
- A measure of the patients perception of severity at discharge (if appropriate)
- The patients perception of the service, its acceptability and quality
- Professional Body / National organisation standards – level of achievement
- Work absence and/or status
- The proportion of out-patient referrals that proceed to surgery
- The impact made on the workload of others
- The impact made on the working lives / CPD of physiotherapists
- Re-referral rate
- Consider following patients up to provide a longer term view

Referral tool

Expressing annual referral rates as a proportion per 1000 of the population

Calculate your present referral rate as an expression of the annual rate per 1000 of the population you serve.

Population = 5000
Total number of referrals per annum = 280 (5000/1000/280)
Referral rate = 56/1000.

Patient self-referral anticipated referral rate calculator

- First, calculate your present referral rate as an expression of the annual rate per 1000 of the population you serve.
- Classify the population in terms of its location, i.e. use national definitions: *urban, semi-rural, rural*. (Non-physiotherapy professions should now seek similar information from their professional contacts or networks. Physiotherapy services can proceed as outlined below.)
- Compare your present rate of referral with the mean according to the classification of location.
- If your referral rate per 1000 is much *lower*, you may anticipate that you will experience an increase in the total number of referrals if you introduce self-referral. However, if the present referral rate per 1000 is *similar* or *exceeds* that quoted, you may anticipate that there will no increase in the number of referrals.

Four abstracts

Abstract 1

Holdsworth L, Webster V and McFadyen A (2004) Direct access to physiotherapy in primary care: now – and into the future? *Physiotherapy*. **90**: 64–72.

Background: Patient direct access to physiotherapy (self-referral) is not the routine mechanism in use within the NHS, although more recently it has become a topic of considerable UK and international interest.

Aim: To develop, implement, investigate and report on a direct access primary care-based physiotherapy service.

Design of Study: Experimental and qualitative.

Setting: A general practice in a health district of Scotland.

Method: The service was introduced and compared to the existing system of open access over a 12-month period. Demographic and clinical data were collected relating to two samples: 'Control Year Group': All general practitioner referrals in the year prior to the study year; 'Study Year Group': general practitioner and direct access referrals. All patients were followed up one month after discharge, and the number of associated general practitioner consultations collated together with clinician views of physiotherapy generally and direct access specifically.

Results: The Control Year and Study Year groups were homogenous with regard to number of referrals (339 vs. 340), patient age, gender, condition category and its severity. There were, however, significant differences between direct-access and general practitioner referrals (22.4% n=76; vs. 77.6% n=264). Direct-access patients were more likely to have been: male, younger, suffering from conditions of a shorter duration, in paid employment with less work absence, more compliant with attendance, had fewer physiotherapy contacts, lower reporting of symptom severity at discharge and were more highly satisfied with their physiotherapy care and experienced fewer general practitioner consultations (p<0.001). Support for direct access was strongly expressed by service users and clinicians.

Conclusions: Direct access to physiotherapy is an example of innovative primary care service provision that is feasible, acceptable to both users and providers, and has major implications for general practitioner workload. Its efficacy, however, should be evaluated in a range of settings before being universally introduced.

Abstract 2

Holdsworth L, Webster V and McFadyen AK (2006a) Self-referral to physiotherapy: deprivation and geographical setting: is there a relationship? Results of a national trial. *Physiotherapy*. **92**: 16–25.

Objectives: To establish the level of self-referral in urban, semi-rural and rural primary care settings that also include a range of deprivation found in Scotland.

Design of Study: Quasi-experimental.

Setting: Twenty-nine general practices throughout Scotland.

Participants: 3010 patients (>16 yrs) and physiotherapists from throughout Scotland

Method: Practices were classified in terms of their location and level of deprivation (DEPCAT). Historical data were used to establish national referral rates in these settings. Self-referral was introduced in each setting and the proportions of patients referring themselves or being referred by their GP were collated over a full year. A further category of 'GP suggested' was also included.

Results: There were different rates of referral according to setting (p<0.001). A national adult referral rate of 53.5/1000 was identified. Rural areas experienced the highest rates (66/1000) compared to 44.5/1000 found in urban and 49/1000 in semi-rural settings. An overall 'true' self-referral rate of 21.5% was found. Rural areas experienced the highest level of both self and GP suggested referral (31.6% and 26%). An increase in total referral numbers was experienced in <20% of locations after introducing self-referral, all of whom had a history of under-provision. Self-referrers came from the range of socio-economic settings included although there were differences observed between the groups (p<0.001).

Conclusions: Introducing self-referral does not appear to result in an increase in the overall referral rate when reasonable levels of service are already being provided in line with national rates according to geographical setting. Deprivation would also appear not to exert a major influence on referral rates. The rate of self-referral into the future, however, is impossible to predict.

Abstract 3

Holdsworth L, Webster V and McFadyen A (2006b) Are patients who refer themselves to physiotherapy different from those referred by GPs? Results of a national trial. *Physiotherapy*. **92**: 26–33.

Objectives: To establish if there are differences in the profile of patients who refer themselves to physiotherapy compared with those referred by or at the suggestion of their GP in a range of primary care settings.

Design of Study: Quasi-experimental.

Setting: Twenty-nine general practices throughout Scotland.

Participants: 3010 patients (>16 ys) and 100 physiotherapists.

Method: Self-referral was introduced in each site. The demographic and clinical data relating to all referrals collated over a full year were compared by referral group: self-referral (SR), GP-suggested (GPS) and GP (GP) referral groups.

Results: There was no relationship between gender or age group and referral group but other differences in the profile were found. The groups differed in terms of their presenting condition and its severity (p=0.027). Greater proportions of GPS and SR patients presented with low back and neck conditions (54% vs. 42.5%, p<0.001). SR patients reported having their symptoms for less than 14 days to a greater extent than the other groups (14% vs. 8.5% and 10%, p=0.011). Non-preferential treatment waiting time to physiotherapy also differed with 44% of SRs being seen within two weeks of referral compared to 35.5% of GPs (p<0.001). SRs were absent from work in lower proportions, 19.5% compared to 27.5% of the other groups (p=0.048) and were absent for half the mean time (2.5 days vs. 6 days). They also completed their treatment in greater proportions (76% vs. 68.5% and 71.5%; p=0.002). Although all groups experienced the same mean number of physiotherapy contacts (4), GPSs had a proportionally lower contact rate with 64.5% having 4 or less contacts compared with 54.5% of SRs and 51% of GP referrals (p<0.001). There was no difference in the outcome determined by either physiotherapist or patient.

Conclusions: Both SRs and GPSs appear to have a different profile from that of GP referrals.

Abstract 4

Holdsworth L, Webster V and McFadyen A (2006) What are the costs to NHS Scotland of self-referral to physiotherapy? Results of a national trial. *Physiotherapy*. (2006) doi: 10.1016/j.physio.2006.05.005.

Background: Recent healthcare policies have encouraged an increasing interest in the concept of patient self-referral, specifically with regard to physiotherapy. What has not been known until recently, however, is the efficacy of this mode of access within the NHS, including the cost implications on which to reliably base the provision of future service models.

Aim: To establish the costs to NHS Scotland of differing modes of access to physiotherapy in primary care.

Design of Study: Cost minimisation analysis, multi-centred national trial.

Setting: Twenty-six general practices throughout Scotland.

Participants: 3010 patients.

Method: Self-referral was introduced in each site in parallel to GP referral. NHS associated cost data was collated over a full year by referral type group, self-referral (SR), GP-suggested (GPS) and GP (GP) referral groups. A cost minimisation analysis was carried out and the main outcome measures were the number of GP and physiotherapy contacts, prescribing of NSAIDs and analgesics, referral for X-ray, MRI and/or to secondary care. Costs were established for 2004.

Results: The data from 3010 patients identified significant associations between referral group and prescribing, referral for X-ray and to secondary care, GP and physiotherapy contacts ($p<0.001$). The average cost of an episode of care was established: £66.31 (SR); £79.50 (GPS); and £88.99 (GP). Extrapolated to identify national implications, the average cost benefit to NHS Scotland was identified as being approximately £2 million per annum.

Conclusion: There are significant positive implications associated with self-referral to physiotherapy which represent added value for NHS Scotland that are also of relevance to the rest of the NHS in the UK.

Glossary

- **Acute sector** Term that is changing in use, but generally describes hospital-based health services which are provided on an inpatient or outpatient basis.
- **Algorithms** Any computation, formula, survey or look-up table that is useful in healthcare, and whose purpose is to improve the delivery of healthcare (www.medalreg.com/www/ftp/amia2002.ppt).
- **Allied health professions (AHP)** Formerly known as the 'professions allied to medicine' (PAM), these healthcare professions (all registered with the Health Professions Council) contribute to both health and social care delivery directly, at any given point of a patient pathway. There are diverse groups under this banner, including art therapists, chiropodists and podiatrists, dieticians, drama therapists, occupational therapists, physiotherapists, prosthetists and orthotists, music therapists, speech and language therapists, and radiographers.
- **Assessment** The clinical process of identifying patients' needs, problems, clinical signs and symptoms.
- **Autonomous practice** The freedom to practise independently of external controls, with increased accountability for the management of patients.
- **Catchment area** The population which lives within a specified geographical area with clearly defined boundaries.
- **Centralised booking system** A means of organising patients' admission to healthcare services. In any booked system the patient is given the choice of when to attend. In a partial booking system the patient is given an indication of how long the wait will be and is contacted by the healthcare provider at some point after the decision to admit, to be given a choice of dates for admission.
- **Clinical audit** A quality improvement process that seeks to improve patient care and outcomes through systematic review of care against explicit criteria and the implementation of chance (NICE, 2004).
- **Clinical governance** 'A framework through which NHS organisations are accountable for continually improving the quality of their services and safeguarding high standards of care by creating an environment in which excellence in clinical care will flourish.' (Scally G and Donaldson LJ (1998) Clinical governance and the drive for quality improvement in the new NHS in England. *BMJ*. **317**(7150): 61–5.)

In Wales, the Welsh Assembly has issued guidance and a review of clinical governance (www.wales.nhs.uk/publications/clinical-governance.pdf).

In Northern Ireland, the Department of Health has established a local clinical and social care governance support team. Published guidelines for implementation may be found at www.dhsspsni.gov.uk/hss/governance/guidance.asp.

NHS Quality Improvement Scotland has a remit to set standards, monitor performance and provide advice, guidance and support to NHS Scotland on effective clinical practice and service improvements (including the implementation of clinical governance) (www.nhshealthquality.org/nhsqis/nhsqis_sub_home.jsp).

- **Clinical guidelines** 'Systematically developed statements to assist practitioner and patient decisions about appropriate healthcare for specific clinical circumstances.' (Field MJ and Lohr KN (1992) *Guidelines for Clinical Practice: from development to use.* National Academic Press, Washington.)
- **Critical friends** Individuals who have the following characteristics: influence; an interest in innovation; and are focused on improving the patient experience, meeting organisational objectives and are fairly senior in their organisation.
- **Critical thinking** The ability to synthesise information, conclusions and points of view clearly, accurately and relevantly. Critical thinking is applied to reading and writing as well as to speaking and listening.
- **Data definitions** A term used to describe the characteristics of each data item. The definition should be strictly adhered to.
- **Data item** An individual piece of information.
- **Dataset** A pre-determined or agreed collection of data items.
- **Diagnosis** The skill and process of distinguishing one disease from another: essential to scientific and successful treatment. Also, the opinion arrived at on the nature of a disease.
- **Duty of care** Ensuring that therapeutic intervention is intended to be of benefit to the patient.
- **Evidence-based practice** Conscientious, explicit and judicious use of current best evidence when making decisions about the care of patients. Practically, it means integrating individual clinical expertise with the best available external clinical evidence from systematic research.
- **Extended scope practitioner (ESP)** 'Extended scope' practitioners are clinical allied health professional specialists in any recognised specialty with an extended scope of practice. This implies working beyond the recognised scope of practice; for example, requesting or undertaking investigations (X-rays, scans, blood tests and so on), using the results of investigations to assist clinical diagnosis and appropriate management of patients, listing for surgery or referring to other medical and healthcare professionals.

- **Face to face** Direct contact between the therapist and patient, as opposed to telephone or written contact.
- **First point of contact practitioner** A healthcare practitioner who is able by professional regulation to be the first point of contact for a patient seeking advice or treatment for a health-related concern.
- **General practitioner (GP)** A medical general practitioner who has, to date, been the gatekeeper to healthcare for patients based in a local community.
- **Health improvement** *England* Before devolution 'health improvement' was a term promoted by the government in the White Paper of July 1999, *Saving Lives: Our Healthier Nation*, which was an action plan to tackle poor health. The objective was to 'improve the health of everyone and the health of the worst-off in particular'. Currently, health improvement is driven by key targets, published by the governments of each of the four UK nations. In England, primary care organisations (known as 'trusts') create local development plans which set out the priorities for health improvement.

  Northern Ireland Each of the four health and social services boards has set up an investing for health partnership at local level and developed a long term local health improvement plan for the implementation of the investing for health strategy.

  Scotland Health improvement has featured strongly in the Scottish Executive policy for health. The Scottish Executive Partnership Agreement states, 'Improving Scotland's health is central to the welfare of our society. Our poor health record is well known. New initiatives are required to create a step change in improving health'. (For the Partnership Agreement, *see* www.scotland.gov.uk/library5/government/pfbs-033.asp).

  Wales There is a statutory duty on local health boards and local authorities to work in partnership to develop a health, social care and well-being strategy based on a local needs assessment.

  All these themes are developed from the 2003 White Paper, *Partnership for Care* (www.scotland.gov.uk/library5/health/pfcs-00.asp).
- **Healthcare practitioner** A person registered with the United Kingdom Central Council for Nursing, Midwifery and Health Visiting (UKCC) or Health Professionals Council (HPC) to work in a specific health discipline.
- **Informed consent** A process through which a patient learns about their potential intervention and management, including the potential risks and benefits, before deciding whether or not to proceed.
- **Information management and technology (IMT)** Also known as 'health informatics': the knowledge, skills and tools which enable information to be collected, managed, used and shared to support the delivery of healthcare and to promote health.

- **Impact** The extent to which outcomes affect overall objectives; may relate to individuals, services and organisations.
- **Monitoring** Collecting information on clinical and non-clinical performance; it may be continuous or intermittent. It may also be undertaken in relation to specific incidents or concerns, or to check key performance areas.
- **Multi-professional team** A group of people from different professions (both healthcare and social care), who work together to provide care for patients with a particular condition. The composition of the team will vary according to different factors, including the patient's condition, the scale of the service being provided and geographical or socioeconomic elements.
- **NHS** National Health Service.
- **Outcome measure** 'A test or scale administered and interpreted by therapists that has been shown to measure accurately a particular attribute of interest to patients and therapists, and is expected to be influenced by intervention.' (Finch E, Brooks, D, Statford PW and Mayo NE (2002) *Physical Rehabilitation Outcome Measures* (2e). Lippincott, Williams and Williams, Canada.)
- **Open access** A system of access to healthcare services used primarily by GPs, but also used by other healthcare professionals, whereby patients are referred to a service for assessment and/or treatment.
- **Pathway** The patient's journey as he or she comes into contact with health and social care services. The term may be applied loosely to describe the options available or more formally where identified, documented pathways are in place. 'Integrated care pathways' are both a tool and a concept, and these embed guidelines, protocols and locally agreed evidence-based, patient-centred best practice into everyday use for individual patients. Integrated care pathways also record deviations from planned care in the form of 'variances'. An integrated care pathway is aimed at having the right people, at the right time, in the right place, with the right outcome – all with attention to the patient's experience and to compare planned care with that actually received.
- **Patient** A person with injury, physical or mental disorder, disease or abnormality who comes into the care of a health practitioner or institution responsible for providing care to such people. Patients are sometimes referred to as 'users' or 'clients'.
- **Patient journey** *See* **Pathway**.
- **Patient self-referral** Patients to refer themselves directly to healthcare providers without having to be seen or prompted by another healthcare practitioner to do so. Self-referral relates to telephone, electronic technology or face-to-face services. Sometimes referred to as 'direct access'.
- **Peer review** Evaluation of the clinical reasoning about a patient episode by a peer at a similar clinical level using patient case notes to guide the discussion. Practitioners should select their own peer(s) and the process is

carried out informally. Peer review tends to have a narrower professional focus than clinical supervision. It is also a process whereby research is scrutinised by experts who have not been involved in its design or execution.

- **Plain English**   A campaign that encourages organisations to use simple, understandable language for public information. Plan English is defined as 'language that the intended audience can understand and act upon from a single reading'. (*See* www.en.wikipedia.org/wiki/Plain_English.)
- **Primary care**   The conventional first point of contact between a patient and the NHS. The component of care delivered to patients outside hospitals and typically, though by no means exclusively, delivered through general practices. Primary care services are the most frequently used of all services provided by the NHS. Primary care encompasses a range of family health services provided by family doctors, dentists, pharmacists, optometrists and ophthalmic medical practitioners.
- **Private therapy practitioner**   A therapist (*see* **Therapist**) who works independently of publicly funded healthcare systems.
- **Professional body**   An organisation, usually non-profit-making, existing to further a particular profession to protect both the public interest and the interests of professionals. These organisations act to protect the public by maintaining and enforcing standards of training and ethics in their professions.
- **Protocol**   Detailed description of the steps taken to deliver care or treatment, or a clinical intervention, in specific circumstances, to a patient. This is sometimes called an 'integrated care pathway'. Protocols may be endorsed nationally or locally.
- **Quality assurance**   Improving performance and preventing problems through planned and systematic activities, including documentation, training and review.
- **Rationale**   The scientific or objective reason for taking a specific action.
- **Referral**   The process whereby a patient is transferred from one professional to another, usually for specialist advice, treatment or both.
- **Scope of practice**   Activities that a profession can or cannot do, set and regulated by professional bodies.
- **Secondary care**   Care provided in an acute sector setting. (*See* **Acute Sector.**)
- **Service user**   *See* **Patient**.
- **Stakeholder**   An individual or group with an interest in the success or a service or organisation in delivering intended results and maintaining the viability of the organisation's services. Stakeholders influence programmes, products and services.
- **Therapist**   A qualified healthcare practitioner who is registered to practise by the Health Professions Council and is either an art therapist, dietician, drama therapist, music therapist, occupational therapist,

optometrist, orthotist, podiatrist, physiotherapist, prosthetist, radiographer or speech and language therapist.

- **Triage** The assessment of patients in order to establish the nature and severity of their healthcare problem. It may lead to a number of options which could include immediate or delayed referral to another healthcare profession, treatment or being placed on a waiting list for future intervention or discharge.
- **Whole-time equivalent (WTE)** A figure used to quantify staffing levels in terms of whole-time equivalents. WTEs are usually reported as a percentage.

Index